YOUR COMPLETE GUIDE TO

Facial Cosmetic Surgery

JON MENDELSOHN, M.D.

WILLIAM TRUSWELL, M.D.

KRISTON KENT, M.D.

Addicus Books
Omaha, Nebraska

AN ADDICUS NONFICTION BOOK

ISBN# 1-886039-70-4

Cover design by Peri Poloni, www.knockoutbooks.com
Interior design by Melissa Marquardt, www.abacusgraphics.com

This book is not intended to serve as a substitute for a physician.
Nor is it the authors' intent to give medical advice contrary to that of an attending physician.

We wish to thank the following corporations for providing photos:
Inamed Aesthetics, Inc., collagen products (Cosmoderm, Cosmoplast, Hylaform) photos, pages 77, 80-84.
Atrium Medical Corp, Advanta facial implants photo, page 80.
S. Jezerinac, Custom Medical Stock Photo, chemical peel application, page 114.
DermaMed USA, Inc., microdermabrasion photo, page 125.

Library of Congress Cataloging-in-Publication Data

Mendelsohn, Jon, 1966-
    Your complete guide to facial cosmetic surgery / Jon Mendelsohn, William Truswell, Kriston Kent.
        p. cm.
    Includes index.
    ISBN 1-886039-70-4 (alk. paper)
1. Surgery, Plastic--Popular works. I. Kent, Kriston, 1959- II. Truswell, William, 1946- III. Title.

RD119.M48 2004
617.5'20592--dc22

2004015459

Addicus Books, Inc.
P.O. Box 45327
Omaha, Nebraska 68145
www.AddicusBooks.com

Printed in the United States of America
10 9 8 7 6 5 4 3 2 1

CONTENTS

· ·

ACKNOWLEDGMENTS

The support and love of many people have helped make this book possible. I would like to thank my wonderful family for all of the support and love they share with me. Of course, the love and magic of living is valued every day as I embrace the life and the joy that Hanny and Benny bring to me every day.

I would also like to extend my sincere thanks and gratitude to my outstanding family of associates that I have been fortunate enough to work with daily. Their dedication to our vision and our patients are second to none. Their tireless efforts are recognized and greatly appreciated. Thank You.

Finally, I would like to thank all of the patients to whom I have been fortunate enough to meet. Every day I receive tremendous satisfaction in knowing that the relationships I have developed with you will last a lifetime. I enjoy educating and being educated by you, and hope that I can continue to provide care to you for years to come.

Jon Mendelsohn, M.D.

The progress of this project has been aided by the support and patience of many whom I hold close in both my personal and professional life. To them I owe a debt of gratitude and to them I offer this book in dedication. Thank you, Lynn, wife, partner, and friend of infinite patience and understanding, for helping keep this tempest in me somewhat near the ground. And to you, Jason and Jody, my now grown children, you who are the brightness and future, thank you.

Thank you, Laura, Kathy, Lisa, Johanne, Cozette, Nancy, Darci, and Jessica, my most wonderful staff, for your loyalty, dedication, hard work, and affection—without you, my practice would be diminished. I also wish to acknowledge the American Academy of Facial Plastic and Reconstructive Surgery, the resource for education, guidance, support, and fraternity for Facial Plastic Surgeons throughout the world.

I also wish to thank Mary Campbell for her editorial support on this project.

William Truswell, M.D.

I would like to thank my wife, Charlotte, and my three wonderful children, Kristi, Allen, and Aimee, for their patience and support of my many professional and educational endeavors. I acknowledge Mary Campbell for her editorial help with this book. I would also like to thank my executive assistant, Lesley Coleman, for all her assistance in making my contributions to this book possible.

Kriston J. Kent, M.D.

INTRODUCTION

*A*t no other time in history have we seen so much media attention focused on cosmetic surgery. We see cosmetic surgical makeovers on national television. We watch programs about cosmetic surgery for movie stars. We read magazines and newspapers, brimming with information about the latest cosmetic surgery techniques and procedures. Why is all this media attention occurring? It's likely due to the public's intense interest in these topics.

Millions of Americans are seeking facial cosmetic surgery. The number of facelifts performed in the United States increased 46 percent over last year. Other procedures, such as rhinoplasty and eyelid lifts, have also increased dramatically. No doubt, part of the upward trend is a result of our population getting older— someone turns 50 every 8 seconds in America. We may be aging, but we want to look our best. Even so, the trends show that many younger Americans are also undergoing cosmetic surgery, too.

Perhaps you're considering facial cosmetic surgery. If so, we encourage you to become an informed consumer so you will enjoy the process and achieve the results you desire. To help you better understand facial cosmetic surgery, we offer descriptions of various procedures along with dozens of before and after photos of our patients. We hope this book is a helpful tool to you as you make choices about facial cosmetic surgery.

CHAPTER 1

CONTEMPLATING FACIAL COSMETIC SURGERY

CONTEMPLATING FACIAL COSMETIC SURGERY

*A*re you among the thousands of Americans who are thinking about facial cosmetic surgery? Have you wondered how you might look after a facelift…a nose job…an eyelid lift? Are you brimming with energy on the inside but showing your age on the outside? If so, facial cosmetic surgery may be for you. Each year, more and more Americans are choosing to turn back the clock with cosmetic surgery.

Before we discuss the most common procedures, let's take a look at why our facial skin and tissues age. Not only will this help you understand how facial structure changes with age, but also it will give you insights about lifestyle habits that can help you maintain the results of cosmetic surgery procedures.

How Facial Structure Changes

Why does facial skin eventually start to droop? Consider this analogy: If you've ever had a lined coat or jacket cleaned, you may have found that the lining shrank during dry cleaning or laundering, making the outer fabric sag. Think of your facial skin as the outer fabric and your bones and supporting tissues as the lining. As those bones and tissues shrink and your muscles lose volume and tone, the skin slips downward, sometimes drooping much as your jacket's outer fabric drapes over the hemline.

Beneath your skin, the SMAS—short for *superficial musculoaponeurotic system*—also begins to sag and droop. Here come jowls, low brows, and other unwanted folds. The SMAS is the curtain of muscles of facial expression and the surrounding connective tissue. As the SMAS descends, the skin becomes less taut.

Layers of fat, called fat pads, under the eyes and under the skin on our cheeks also keep us looking younger. When gravity pulls at the cheek pads, it can create sagging skin and hollows under the eyes; it also deepens the nasolabial folds, the grooves that run from both sides of the nose to the corners of the mouth. As the cheek pads get longer, they become less rounded, the face appears flatter, and their weight pulls down the corners of the mouth. As muscles surrounding the eyes shrink and weaken, they sometimes develop small gaps through which fat protrudes, creating little bumps under the eyes.

In addition to changes in the underlying structures of the face, the skin itself changes. We start seeing broken capillaries, rough patches, discolorations, fine lines, and enlarged pores.

Why Skin Ages
Slowing Metabolism

Over the years your *metabolic rate*—the pace at which your body absorbs and processes nutrients—gets slower. As a result your system produces less of just about everything, including blood, bone, the skin proteins *collagen* and elastin, and natural skin oils. Skin-cell growth and replacement also slow down.

As the connective tissues in your body weaken, your skin's support structure is undermined. With less *collagen*, which acts as a glue to hold tissues together, and *elastin*, the fibrous protein in elastic tissues, your skin starts to lose its snap, kind of like an elastic waistband after years of wear. When you were younger, your skin bounced back from all types of stresses, but as the calendar pages flew by, so did your skin's resilience.

Sun Damage

Compare the skin on the underside of your arm to that on the front. That's one way to see how the sun damages your skin. The skin on your under arm is white and unflawed, but the skin on the front of your arm is darker and has been affected by the sun. In fact, you've been bombarded for years with the sun's *ultraviolet alpha*

> *It's important that patients realize that plastic surgery is about "improvement" and not "perfection." The benefits should be increased self-esteem and confidence that allows each patient to have more meaningful relationships at home, work, and with themselves.*
>
> — *Dr. Jon Mendelsohn*

> *The best facial cosmetic-surgery candidates are healthy, active people who really love life and who basically see themselves as looking ten to fifteen years older than the person inside.*
>
> — *Dr. Kriston Kent*

and *beta waves (UV-A* and *UV-B rays)*; the more time you've spent in the sun, the more your unprotected skin has been injured.

UV-A and UV-B rays are responsible for *photoaging*—sun-induced skin damage. UV rays are more harmful at high altitudes, in the summer, and closer to the equator. The sun causes almost as much damage as your biological clock does, sometimes more. Sunlight on unprotected skin penetrates several layers to stimulate pigment-producing *melanin*, which protectively comes to the surface and makes you tan or freckle. Tanned skin filters out some of the UV rays, but harmful amounts still get through. And over time those cute freckles may turn into liver spots, sun spots, or age spots.

Repeated sun exposure, beginning in childhood, accumulates to break down collagen and elastin, worsening wrinkles and fine lines. Sun exposure also breaks down blood vessels, resulting in spider veins. If you haven't protected your eyes properly, you may also have permanent squint lines.

You might see pink scaley lesions on your skin called *actinic keratoses*—small, hardened areas of sun-damaged skin that are often precancerous. Since sun exposure is the number one cause of skin cancer, ask your doctor about any peculiar or unexplained blemishes, especially if they grow or change shape.

Genetics

You have a lot to thank your parents and grandparents for, including your facial bone structure, skin thickness and tone, and pigmentation. These ancestors may have passed along other factors that affect your skin, such as a tendency to gain weight or a medical condition such as hypothyroidism, which often dries out the skin.

Poor Nutrition and Hygeine

Nutrition plays a big role in the condition of your skin. The condition of your skin and hair can testify to this. A poor diet, inadequate fluid intake, and substance abuse are reflected in the appearance of your skin. The longer harmful habits continue, the greater the damage they cause to skin and overall health. Obesity can affect how early and how severely your face loses its youthful firmness. Not only is there more fat to slide into your chin and neck, but every time you lose weight only to gain it back, your skin becomes a bit more slack.

Proper cleansing and moisturizing of the skin is important, also. Too little hygiene is bad for the skin; similarly, over cleansing can remove natural oils, which is damaging to the skin.

Inadequate Sleep

Your body is rejuvenated every time you sleep, repairing the physical insults and psychological strains of the day. Tissues need a hiatus during which they, like you, get a new lease on life. Thus, chronic lack of sleep is a key contributor to premature aging.

Illness and Injury

Injuries and skin disorders such as acne and herpes can leave the face scarred and the features uneven. Chronic illnesses and long-term stress rob your skin of nutrients, especially when accompanied by inadequate self-care. Many medications and topical creams can also deplete nutrients, usually by making your skin more sensitive to the sun. The antibiotic tetracycline, the pain-reliever naproxen (Aleve), and skin-smoothing retinoids (such as Retin-A™ and Renova™) are just a few examples of sun-sensitizers, which make you more prone to sunburn and resulting sun-damaged skin.

Use of Facial Muscles

You've heard of laugh lines, frown lines, even smile lines. Smiling and laughing are much more beneficial than harmful to your health, but repeated facial expression eventually can create lines and wrinkles.

Smoking

Smoking, besides etching vertical wrinkles around your mouth, causes biochemical changes in skin tissues. Cigarette chemicals, when inhaled, constrict small blood vessels so fewer nutrients and less oxygen find their way to skin cells. Smoking also accelerates the aging process and interferes with healing, which is all important after plastic surgery.

Toxins and Irritants

A variety of toxins and irritants can affect the health of your skin. Like excess sunlight and smoking, such things as alcohol and air pollution affect your skin. How so? They stimulate free radicals, which are oxygen molecules that have become unstable. These unstable molecules may then attach to tissues such as collagen in the skin, causing damage. Overtime, this can cause the skin to lose elasticity and become discolored and wrinkled.

Fortunately, the body has defenses, called antioxidants, that fight free radicals. Vitamins C, D, and E are also thought to prevent free radicals from harming tissues. Selenium and green tea are also considered antioxidants.

Is Cosmetic Surgery for You?

If you want to look younger and more radiant, or improve a facial feature you're self-conscious about, you are probably a candidate for facial cosmetic surgery. In fact, most healthy adults could benefit from one or more procedures. Dramatic improvement is possible for men and women in their thirties to their seventies and even eighties, regardless of skin color, skin tone, or bone structure.

The best candidates for facial cosmetic surgery have realistic expectations, are well informed about the procedure, and are in good physical and emotional health.

Attitude and Expectations

Cosmetic surgeons will tell you that your expectations and attitude are the most important qualifications. If you like yourself and you're seeking improvement, not perfection, you'll most likely be pleased with the results of your surgery. Most patients experience enhanced self-confidence and a sense of well-being. Facial rejuvenation can make you look younger, but feeling younger comes only from good health. And although a more youthful appearance can boost your confidence and self-esteem, cosmetic surgery itself cannot make you happy if you are basically unhappy. If you are depressed or your life is a mess, you should probably postpone cosmetic surgery until you feel more stable emotionally.

When Cosmetic Surgery Might Not Be for You

If your goals are realistic, there could be yet other reasons that you are not a good candidate for surgery. Some chronic health conditions may mean that cosmetic surgery should wait. Examples of such health conditions include: uncontrolled high blood pressure; blood disorders, such as excessive bleeding or clotting, or a family history of blood disorders; a history of hypertrophic or keloid scars (types of severe scarring); connective-tissue disorders; heart, lung, kidney, or liver disease; long-term steroid use or use of other drugs (such as Accutane™ for acne) that can interfere with healing; endocrine disorders of the thyroid, parathyroid, or adrenal glands; diabetes; osteoporosis or another bone disorder; autoimmune disease, such as lupus or rheumatoid arthritis; and obesity or anorexia.

Overweight patients may need to take off pounds and stabilize their weight before surgery, and smokers will have to quit, at least for several weeks before and after the operation. The surgeon will caution patients with thicker skin that they might scar heavily.

If, in spite of a medical condition, you are committed to having facial plastic surgery, ask your doctor to recommend treatments or regimens that can make you a better candidate and probably a healthier human being as well.

What's the Next Step?

Arrange a consultation with an experienced, well-qualified facial plastic surgeon. Most patients, doctors report, are pleased with the growing range of treatment choices in facial plastic surgery. Many cosmetic surgeons urge prospective patients to become well informed. The best patients, they say, are those who understand how skin damage and wear occur, how cosmetic procedures can help, and why some people are better candidates for surgery than others.

CHAPTER 2

CHOOSING A FACIAL COSMETIC SURGEON

CHOOSING A FACIAL COSMETIC SURGEON

hoosing a highly qualified, experienced facial plastic surgeon is the single most important thing you can do to ensure that your surgery is a success. Do your homework to find the right one. Ask for referrals from your family doctor, friends, relatives, your hair stylist, and your cosmetologist; however, don't rely completely on even the warmest recommendation. Learn all you can about the surgeon you're considering. Call the doctor's office and ask questions. Visit the doctor's Web site. Ideally, you would interview everyone you're considering; however, note that most facial plastic surgeons charge a fee for a prospective patient consultation.

Surgeon Qualifications

The most important qualifications for a facial plastic surgeon are rigorous training, ample experience, board certification, demonstrated excellence, and compatibility. How can you tell if you and a particular doctor are compatible? Trust your instincts, but also try to judge whether he or she will patiently answer all your questions, treat you as an equal, willingly show you patients' before-and-after pictures, and give you names of former patients to contact.

How Much Experience Is Enough?

Almost all the literature talks about choosing a qualified facial plastic surgeon. Sometimes we are urged to ask a surgeon how many years he or she has been doing surgery, or, for example, how many rhinoplasties the surgeon does each year. However, as prospective patients, most of us do not know what the right answer would be. If a surgeon tells you he or she does 20 rhinoplasties a year or 100, which answer indicates proficiency?

There are no hard and fast numbers to go by here; however, you want to make sure that your surgeon has been trained specifically for the procedure you are considering. Ideally, this highly trained surgeon has been in practice for several years and is performing facial plastic surgery on a regular basis. You're probably in good hands if the doctor is performing the procedure you're considering at least several dozen times a year.

Finally, check to see whether the doctor is certified by organizations such as the American Board of Facial Plastic and Reconstructive Surgery (ABFPRS) or the American Board of Plastic Surgery. Surgeons must meet rigorous standards in both training and experience to be members of these organizations. Other upstanding organizations—known as "societies," "academies," or "colleges"—are typically involved in educational conferences and other continuing education activities; however, the organizations that are "boards" are the ones involved in certifying surgeons. (The Resources section, toward the end of this book, tells you how to contact these and other helpful organizations.)

When you're in the hands of a well-qualified surgeon, you will almost certainly achieve good or excellent results with very little risk. Still, remember that many cosmetic procedures are relatively new and involve important facial muscles and nerves. Make sure your chosen doctor has performed your intended procedure a great many times and kept up with advances in the field. Also, be aware that in many states any licensed physician can perform cosmetic surgery and legally claim to be a facial plastic surgeon.

It is critical that you do enough research—read books, search the Web, and conduct phone and office interviews, for example—to choose the right facial plastic surgeon.

When choosing a doctor, experience counts. It takes a long time to build a reputation for excellence in cosmetic surgery.

— Dr. William Truswell

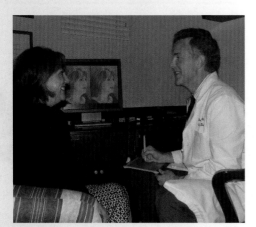

This woman is considering an endoscopic fore-head lift. During her consultation, Dr. Kriston Kent uses on-screen photos of her face to simulate the results of the surgery.

Your Consultation

You'll have at least one and maybe two consultations with your surgeon before your procedure. Whether the doctor is one of several you're considering or is the surgeon you've chosen after doing your research, go to the initial visit well prepared. Educate yourself about facial plastic surgery, particularly about the procedure or procedures that interest you. Be prepared to ask questions during your initial consultation. Some individuals are more comfortable if they take a friend or companion along for the consultation. A companion can help you take notes and be sure you've asked all the pertinent questions.

Determining Your Goals

As you contemplate facial cosmetic surgery, your surgeon may tell you about procedures you didn't realize were available. Or you may learn that the procedure you're considering may not do all you thought it would, and you may benefit more from another procedure.

As you contemplate which procedures would be best for you, keep in mind the three basic ways in which aging affects the face: sagging skin, loss of plumpness, and loss of smooth skin texture. Accordingly, three separate types of procedures are used to reduce these signs of aging. Sagging skin is treated by lifting facial skin and tissue. Loss of plumpness is treated with fillers, whether injectable fillers or implants. Skin texture is rejuvenated with skin resurfacing, either by laser or with chemical peels.

During the consultation, the doctor will probably ask what you like and don't like about your appearance, what makes you self-conscious, what you'd like to change, and what you're hoping to look like after surgery. Maybe your ideal is out of reach, but by knowing what you want, your doctor can tell you what can be achieved. What you'll probably discover is that the procedure your doctor recommends can dramatically improve your appearance in ways you might not have envisioned.

He or she will examine your facial features, skin, expressions, and bone structure, and will explain the procedures that would benefit you, along with their risks and side effects. You'll look at before-and-after pictures of other patients who have had the same procedures. The doctor may take a digital photo of you that can be modified on a computer as you discuss your goals and concerns. For example, if you're considering a nose job, the doctor can project a picture of your profile on the computer screen and then digitally shape your nose to give you a better idea of how the proposed changes might look. This tool gives you and the surgeon a way to see the possibilities as well as any limitations of a procedure.

The doctor might recommend additional surgery be done before, after, or at the same time as the primary operation. For example, a facelift alone may not remove some skin flaws such as mottled skin or sun damage. Accordingly, a surgeon might recommend facial skin resurfacing along with the facelift. Or, if you're interested in a nose job and a facelift, the doctor may recommend these procedures be done separately. If you have chosen a skilled and reputable surgeon, he or she will recommend these procedures only if they will help you achieve your goals and for no other reason. As safe and effective as facial cosmetic surgery has proven to be, no surgery is risk free and no ethical surgeon will carelessly expose you to unnecessary risk and prolonged recovery.

Go to the consultation with an open mind. The procedure you've investigated might not be the right one for you. You may have explored eyelid surgery in detail, but the surgeon thinks a browlift is a better way to go. If you trust the doctor, then find out all you can about browlifts.

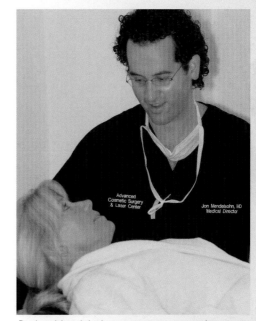

Dr. Jon Mendelsohn answers a patient's questions as she is being prepared for a modified deep chemical peel to eliminate fine wrinkles and improve skin tone.

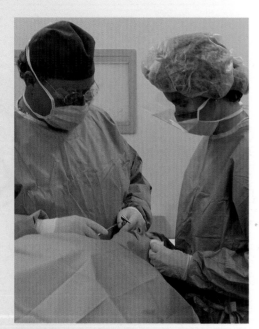

Dr. William Truswell performs a standard SMAS facelift, a procedure that usually takes two to three hours.

What to Take with You

When it comes to your medical history, don't trust your memory. Questions such as "When was your last tetanus shot?" can catch you off guard. If you don't already have copies of all your records, get them and make copies for your doctor. Here's a suggested inventory:

■ Past and current medical conditions, hospitalizations, operations, and noninvasive cosmetic procedures (chemical peels, Botox™, laser resurfacing).

■ Lab work and results of other diagnostic procedures such as CT scans, MRIs, and X-rays.

■ Details about allergies and sensitivities to foods, medicines, soaps, and potential irritants such as adhesive bandages and latex.

■ Drugs you're taking, prescription and nonprescription medications, vitamins and minerals, herbs, and other dietary supplements.

■ Dental history.

■ Eye exam and eye surgery information. Take your eyeglasses and contact lenses to the consultation.

Do not conceal any health information because you think it's unimportant or because it might disqualify you. For example, tell the surgeon if you are currently a smoker. If you do not fully disclose all information, you could be putting yourself at unnecessary risk.

The Surgical Center

Find out where the doctor you're considering performs surgery. Rather than a hospital, the location is more likely to be an outpatient surgery center or the doctor's surgical suite. Ideally, it will be certified as a Medicare Ambulatory Surgery Center or accredited by one of the other nationally recognized oversight organizations; these include the Accreditation Association for Ambulatory Health Care (AAAHC), the American Association for Accreditation of Ambulatory Surgery Facilities (AAAASF), or the Joint Commission for Accreditation of Healthcare Organizations (JCAHO).

Why is accreditation important? It increases the patient's level of safety. If a surgical center has been accredited, it has been inspected for its standard of care and its equipment, including emergency equipment. An accredited center will also have an established relationship with local hospitals and emergency rooms.

Questions to Ask the Surgeon

- What are your medical credentials?
- What procedure or procedures do you recommend for me?
- How many of these procedures have you performed?
- Are there alternatives that might accomplish my goals?
- What are the risks and side effects?
- May I talk to at least one of your patients who has had this procedure?
- Where will the operation be performed?
- How long will the operation take?
- What kind of anesthetic will be used?
- Will I have pain?
- How will I look after surgery?
- How long is the recovery period?
- What kind of postoperative self-care will be necessary?
- When can I go back to work and resume other normal activities?

CHAPTER 3

BEFORE AND AFTER FACIAL COSMETIC SURGERY: WHAT TO EXPECT

BEFORE AND AFTER FACIAL COSMETIC SURGERY: WHAT TO EXPECT

here is more to your summer vacation than the time you spend on the road, in the motel, and at the theme park. It starts months, maybe years, in advance with planning and preparation. Part of the fun is the anticipation. Another part is the experience itself. Finally, there's the transition from the holiday retreat back to the real world.

Likewise, facial cosmetic surgery is more than the time you spend on the operating table. A happy and healthy outcome starts with an idea that takes shape through planning, preparation, and informed choices. It continues through surgery and recovery and culminates in the fulfillment of your hopes and expectations. The best cosmetic procedures, like the best vacations, have lasting value.

Before Your Surgery

At your consultation or at a pre-op teaching visit, your doctor will fill you in on details of the procedure. The topics likely to be covered include:

- Surgical techniques, including incision placement, and objectives

- Side effects and potential risks

- Information about anesthesia, hospital or clinic arrangements, and length of stay

- Pre- and postoperative instructions, including follow-up office visits

- Costs

Arrange for a Caregiver

You'll need to have someone drive you to and from surgery and care for you at home the first day or two. Why do you need a caregiver? You will be groggy from your anesthesia, so you won't be able to drive. Once at home, you may feel a bit weak or your moving about may be restricted. For example, you'll be asked to not bend over or lift. Having a caregiver is so important that the surgeon's office may require that you furnish the name and phone number of your caregiver.

Stop Taking Certain Medications and Supplements

Pain relievers and other medications, vitamins, and herbs that are generally safe may not mix with surgery, the anesthesia, and other medications. Some substances raise your heartbeat or blood pressure, thin your blood so that it doesn't clot normally, or affect the amount of anesthesia needed.

Your doctor will tell you what substances to avoid before surgery and how far in advance to stop using them. Don't assume that something you're taking or plan to take is acceptable just because it isn't on the list. Ask the doctor. Substances that might be off limits include antinausea medications, anti-inflammatory drugs and anything that tends to thin the blood, such as Coumadin; preparations containing aspirin or ibuprofen; supplements that contain vitamin E, ginkgo biloba, ginseng, ginger, echinacea, black cohosh, or other herbs; and red wine and other alcoholic beverages. It's important to give the doctor a *complete* medication and supplement list at your consultation so that he or she will be able to tell you which of those substances to stop taking and what substitutes might be available.

Fill Your Prescriptions

Depending on the procedure and the doctor's preferences, you might be given prescriptions for antibiotics, pain relievers, antihistamines, d............nts, anti-inflammatory drugs, stool softeners, vitamins, ointments, and sedativ.... uch as Valium. The doctor or a highly trained clinic staff member will tell you when tu start and stop taking these prescriptions.

Many cosmetic surgeons are recommending specific preparations of *Arnica montana* and *bromelain*—botanical products that are believed to speed healing. If your doctor doesn't mention these, ask about them.

You might be a bit confused if the surgeon tells you to stop taking your anti-inflammatory medication and then hands you a prescription for an anti-inflammatory drug. Likewise, you may be told to stop taking blood-thinning agents only to have blood thinners given to you before or during surgery. It's important for you to understand that these drugs are safe, effective, and even necessary when the doctor prescribes the specific products and dosages and controls when, where, and how they are used.

Grow Your Hair

If you're having a facelift, a browlift, eyelid surgery, or otoplasty, one of the first things you might want to do before surgery is start growing your hair. Your hair will hide incisions while they're healing, though most incisions are well hidden. Otoplasty patients sometimes prefer not to draw attention to their ears after surgery.

Quit Smoking

If you smoke, you'll need to quit two weeks or more before surgery and remain a nonsmoker throughout your recovery. As smoke enters the bloodstream, it compromises vascular function, interferes with proper healing, and increases the chance for complications. In fact, it is estimated that the risk of skin death, or *necrosis*, is 1,500 percent more likely for smokers than for non-smokers. This applies to all forms of smoking—cigarettes, cigars, and pipes.

Follow Your Diet Instructions

Your surgeon might give you a diet to follow in the weeks before surgery. Dine well the evening before your procedure, because you'll probably be told not to eat or drink anything after midnight except small sips of water needed to swallow medications. Avoid alcohol the evening before surgery because alcohol tends to thin your blood and can lead to increased bruising.

Cleanse Your Hair and Face

You might be instructed to shower and wash your hair with an antiseptic shampoo both the night before and the morning of surgery. In any case, your hair should be clean and free of styling products. After washing your face, don't apply moisturizers or other skin conditioners unless your doctor says it's okay.

It's extremely important to follow your doctor's directions meticulously, for your own safety and for the best possible outcome. Call the office and ask about instructions you don't understand.

At the Surgical Center

Arrive at the surgical facility wearing loose-fitting clothes you can take off and put on without pulling them over your head—a shirt or sweater that fastens up the front, for example. Don't wear makeup, jewelry, or fragrance.

Before the operation, depending on the type of procedure and your doctor's practice, the medical staff will prepare you for surgery.

- You may be given a pill or an injection to help you relax. If not, and you are anxious, ask if you can have a sedative.

- Monitoring pads may be taped to your chest to keep track of your vital signs.

- You may have an IV in place, probably in your arm, delivering saline solution to keep you hydrated, as well as a small plastic port inserted for administering anesthetics, antibiotics, and other medications. Placement of the IV and port won't be painful, though you might feel a slight stinging for a few seconds.

- You'll probably be given IV sedation and local anesthesia, which your doctor may refer to as *twilight sleep* or *managed-care anesthesia*. Local anesthesia with sedation will keep you asleep during surgery. It's unlikely you'll have *general anesthesia* unless you're undergoing additional complex procedures at the same time. General anesthesia puts you into a deep sleep during surgery.

- Your doctor will use a marking pen to mark your face to indicate placement of the incisions.

After Your Surgery

After the operation you'll remain in the recovery room where you'll continue to be monitored in the unlikely event of high blood pressure, bleeding, or reaction to anesthesia. If you feel nauseated, let your attendant know right away and you'll be given antinausea medication.

After an hour or so, when the anesthetic has worn off, and you're fully awake, you can probably go home. Under no circumstances will you be allowed to drive after surgery, so be sure you've arranged for a driver and at-home caregiver. You'll probably leave the recovery room with instructions to rest and let your caregiver prepare meals and assist you with going to the bathroom and other tasks.

You should have little or no pain, but you will be prescribed a prescription pain reliever to use just in case. If you are uncomfortable to the point where you have trouble resting, don't hesitate to take the over-the-counter pain reliever your doctor recommended or the medication he or she prescribed. Sleep and relaxation are essential for healing.

To make sure you're comfortable after surgery and to speed healing, your doctor will give you specific instructions for self-care and a timetable for resuming your usual activities. The instructions depend on several factors: the type of procedure, the approach used, other procedures done at the same time, and your doctor's own experience and preferences.

To speed healing, your surgeon may also use autologous platelet gel during your surgery. This gel is derived from about two ounces of the patient's own blood, drawn during the surgery. The blood is spun through a centrifuge to separate the platelets, which contain bioactive proteins. When applied under a skin flap, the platelet-rich gel helps to seal, repair, and regenerate the tissues disturbed during surgery.

Common Post-Surgical Instructions

- Keep your head elevated. When sleeping, use at least two pillows and try to lie on your back.

- Avoid bending over, lifting, or straining—in short, doing anything that might raise your blood pressure, putting a strain on your healing tissues.

- Use lightweight ice packs as directed to control swelling. You might use soft gel packs, or bags of frozen peas or corn, wrapped in a towel. You may be given a prescription drug to help reduce swelling.

- Care for your incisions may involve changing gauze pads and using a topical antibacterial ointment, such as Bacitracin and hydrogen peroxide. Do not use vitamin E on the incisions.

- Start out with a liquid or soft diet—not too hot or too cold.

- Avoid moving your mouth and facial muscles excessively by chewing, talking, laughing, smiling, drinking through a straw, yawning, even putting on lipstick. You might be advised not to tweeze your eyebrows or wear earrings.

- Stay out of the sun. When your doctor gives the okay, wear sunscreen (at least SPF 15) and a hat with a brim.

- Take prescribed and recommended medications, which may include drugs for pain, stool softeners so you don't have to strain when going to the bathroom, suppositories for nausea, sedatives to help you sleep, antibiotics to prevent infection, vitamins and food supplements, Arnica montana or bromelain for healing, and other products approved by your doctor.

- Avoid aspirin, ibuprofen, vitamin E, and other blood-thinning substances—they may promote bleeding.

- Avoid alcohol as long as you're taking sedatives or pain medications. Your doctor may tell you not to use alcohol for three or four days after surgery, even if you're not taking those drugs.

■ Refrain from smoking and stay away from heavy second-hand smoke for at least two weeks.

■ Protect the surgery area from impact and injury. Wear clothing that doesn't have to be pulled over your head.

Your first follow-up office visit will be a day or two after your surgery. At this appointment or a later one, your doctor will remove drainage tubes (if any) and any bandages. The surgeon will also remove any sutures, skin clips, splints, or packing during surgery.

In the weeks ahead your life will return to normal. Your doctor may give you a specific timetable indicating when you can resume normal activities, such as:

■ Taking a shower

■ Using a hair dryer—probably on the low setting at first

■ Wearing your glasses or contact lenses

■ Brushing your teeth, shaving, putting on makeup

■ Resuming non-strenuous activities

■ Driving a car, which will most likely be when you can turn your head easily

■ Resuming sexual activity

■ Returning to work if it's not physically strenuous

■ Resuming strenuous activities, such as heavy housework and noncontact sports

■ Going swimming

■ Playing contact sports

The better you take care of yourself—following your doctor's instructions to the last detail—the sooner you'll be back in the swing of things and enjoying your younger, fresher look.

Common Side Effects

With each day that passes after surgery, you'll feel more energetic and you'll start to see the benefits of your new look. Healing can be a gradual process, but you can speed it along by following your doctor's instructions and taking as much downtime as he or she recommends. Keep in mind that you may experience some normal side effects as you're healing.

Soreness. Severe pain is unusual after facial cosmetic surgery, but you may feel some stiffness, tenderness, or possibly mild headaches at first. These symptoms can be easily managed with prescription or over-the-counter pain medication. Take only pain relievers prescribed or recommended by your doctor; products containing aspirin or ibuprofen can thin the blood and interfere with healing.

Bruising. You might see temporary bruising, which will fade quickly. Your doctor can recommend camouflage makeup suitable for both men and women.

Swelling. Using ice packs according to your doctor's instructions should keep swelling to a minimum. Bags of frozen vegetables, such as corn or peas wrapped in a towel, work well.

Temporary scarring at the incision lines. Your surgeon will have placed the incisions where scars will be inconspicuous, and they will fade over time, becoming barely visible. In addition, itching, slight bleeding, oozing, and crusting may occur at the incision site. Your doctor will tell you what to expect following your procedure and will tell you how to minimize any side effects.

Low mood. It is not unusual to feel a little down now and then during the first few weeks of the healing phase. Keep in mind why you wanted the procedure and how wonderful you will look very soon. If you're well prepared with ways to entertain yourself and if your emotional health is generally stable, your low mood is unlikely to last. Make arrangements for work and family responsibilities while you recover so you won't lie there fretting about what's not being done. Upbeat books and movies can occupy your mind and lift your mood.

Temporary numbness, loss of sensation. At first, you might experience numbness in the area where incisions were made. This common occurrence is a result of small nerve branches, under the skin, being cut or stretched during a procedure. These nerves should heal, restoring normal sensation to the area. In some cases, numbness may take several months to completely resolve.

Risks and Complications

Millions of Americans have cosmetic plastic surgery each year, and over a third of them are repeat patients who have had other procedures. The majority are pleased with the results and have no lasting complications. Still, as a surgical procedure, these procedures are to be taken seriously, and it's important to understand potential complications.

Infection. Your doctor's expertise and your own self-care, including the antibiotics you'll take before and after surgery, should prevent infection. Let your doctor know right away if there is inflammation, pus, or unusual pain at the incision lines, or if your temperature rises more than one and a half degrees above normal.

Bleeding. If there's any bleeding at all after your procedure, it should be slight and short-lived. More than a little bleeding is unusual and should be reported to your doctor immediately.

Hematoma. A hematoma—a blood-filled swelling under the skin—occurs less than three percent of the time in facial plastic surgery. A tender, raised area filled with fluid can indicate hematoma even if you can't see any blood. If necessary, the doctor can drain a small hematoma with a needle. Large, spreading hematomas require your doctor's immediate attention in order to prevent tissue damage.

Careful surgeons monitor bleeding during the surgery and use techniques that make hematoma formation very unlikely. Some surgeons use a *closed-suction drain*—a small tube under the skin behind the ear. Many doctors, however, are turning to other techniques, such as the use of platelet gel, that not only prevent hematomas but reduce bruising and speed healing.

Seroma. Similar to a hematoma, a seroma is a pool of fluid that forms under the skin; however, the fluid is not blood but a sterile body fluid. Seromas may dissolve on their own, or the doctor may need to drain them with a thin needle. Like hematomas, seromas are less likely to occur with the use of small surgical drains or platelet-rich plasma during surgery.

Incision complications. Rarely, incisions become crusty. In this case, your doctor will give you instructions on how to clean them. Follow the surgeon's advice carefully to promote incision healing. As mentioned earlier, scars may be more noticeable on thicker-skinned patients.

Excessive scarring, such as hypertrophic scars (overdeveloped scars) or keloids along the incision lines, and permanent scarring are rare among patients with no history of scarring problems.

Anesthesia reaction. An allergic reaction to the anesthesia or another medication is usually preventable; your doctor will learn of the possibility while reviewing your medical history and take preventive measures. Such a reaction is rare in any case, especially when sedation and local anesthesia are used. If it does occur, it will probably be observed and treated during recovery at the surgical center or doctor's office.

Other complications. Fewer than one percent of patients experience complications such as nerve or muscle damage leading to numbness and loss of movement. Discuss the risk of such complications with your doctor.

Although it's important to be aware of risks, note that a 2003 study reported that the rate of complications from plastic surgery, whether performed in a hospital or a doctor's accredited surgical suite, was below one percent—significantly lower than for a tonsillectomy. Other studies indicate that most patients are satisfied with their plastic surgery outcomes and enjoy significant improvement in quality of life. For study data, visit the Web sites of the organizations listed in the Resources section at the end of this book.

CHAPTER 4

FACELIFT

4

FACELIFT

*I*t has often been referred to as "bloom"—that fresh, full-cheeked, buoyant face that radiates health and energy. You might still feel like a flower at its glorious best, although your face may have lost its more youthful look. Gravity causes sagging and the years carve lines in cheeks formerly smooth and firm. There may be deepening furrows between your mouth and chin, your jaw line may disappear, and the corners of your mouth might turn down, making you look sad or angry.

If you are unhappy about such signs of aging, you may wish to consider having a facelift. Each year more than one hundred thousand Americans, 90 percent of them women, choose to have facelifts.

What Is a Facelift?

A facelift is a surgical procedure that restores a more youthful and natural look to the face and neck. A facelift smoothes and tightens facial skin, improving the sagging in your cheeks, chin, and neck. A facelift can also lessen the grooves, known as marionette lines, from the corners of your lips to your chin and many of the wrinkles in your neck and the lower part of your face.

Today, facial plastic surgeons use techniques that achieve a natural look, turning the clock back ten years or more and giving you renewed confidence in your appearance. How long will a facelift last? There is no single answer to this question for everyone; however, a facelift may last for five to twelve years. Factors include genetics, of course, along with lifestyle: if you avoid weight gain and loss, don't smoke, and stay out of the sun, your facelift will last longer. Your age when you have a facelift is also a factor. For example, a 40-year-old person will have more skin elasticity than a 70-year-old; therefore, the older person may see new signs of aging sooner than a younger person.

Facelifts have been around in one form or another since the beginning of the twentieth century, mostly as skin-only procedures. In fact, Americans who had facelifts before the 1970s came out of surgery with smoother skin, but often with a stretched, "wind tunnel" look. Not only did these facelifts look artificial, they didn't last as long as today's more sophisticated procedures.

Today, you're likely to hear about numerous kinds of facelifts; however, several types and techniques are popular.

Basic Types of Facelifts

SMAS Facelift

As mentioned earlier, the SMAS refers to the subcutaneous musculoaponeurotic system, which is the curtain of facial muscles that lie under the skin. In the late 1970s, the SMAS facelift became the standard. This procedure tightens the SMAS as well as the skin of the lower part of the face, including the chin and the front of the neck. Because the underlying muscles are also tightened, the SMAS facelift smoothes the skin naturally, avoiding a pulled look. The SMAS facelift does not significantly change nasolabial folds or sagging fat pads under the cheek.

Another procedure, known as an *extended SMAS facelift* goes farther toward the nose to smooth lines around the nose and mouth.

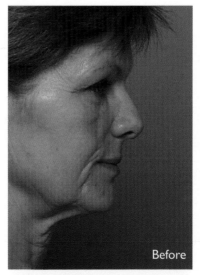
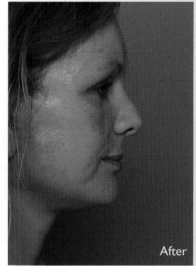
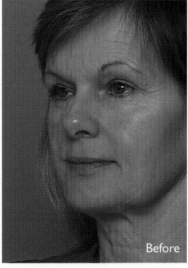
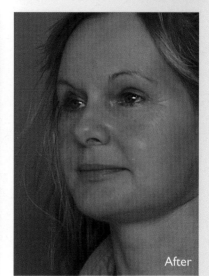

Facelift with endoscopic browlift.

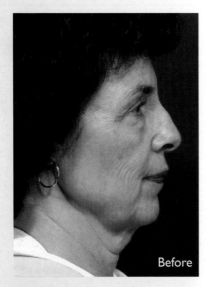

Before

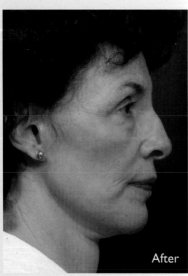

After

Deep-Plane Facelift

Another type of facelift, the *deep-plane facelift* can improve midface drooping and the deep folds running from the cheek to the lip. This facelift differs from the SMAS facelift in that it develops a thicker flap and allows more movement of the mid-cheek tissues. Some surgeons feel they get a more dramatic result that lasts longer with the deep-plane lift. However, some studies have demonstrated no advantage of deep-plane over standard SMAS lifts when patients had alternate sides of their faces done with the different techniques. The deep-plane lift is technically more difficult to perform, it involves greater risk to facial nerves, and it requires much longer recovery than a standard facelift.

There are variations of deep-plane lifts, including a *subperiosteal lift*, which lifts and repositions tissues—skin, fat, and muscle—all at once. Another variation, the *composite facelift*, includes an extra step to include the muscle around the lower eyelid.

Mini Lift

This procedure involves minimal incisions and is best suited for younger patients, perhaps in their 30s or 40s. The procedure can involve skin only, and may not lift the underlying muscle structures. As a result, the procedure does not significantly improve any skin laxity in the neck or jowl area. This type of procedure is sometimes also referred to as a "weekend lift" or an "S-lift," so called for the S-shaped incision made in the hairline. The results of this procedure will not last as long as those in which the underlying muscles are also lifted.

Are You a Candidate for a Facelift?

Almost anyone whose face shows the effects of aging and environmental damage can benefit from a facelift. The procedure is performed with excellent results in both light- and dark-skinned individuals in their thirties to sixties or seventies and even in their eighties if they're in good health. People who are mildly to moderately

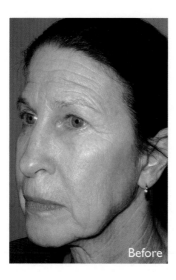
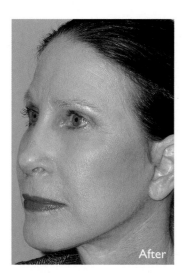

Before

After

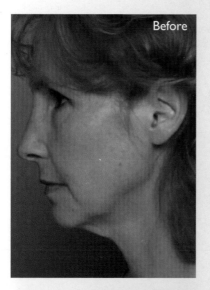

Before

overweight may enjoy some improvement from a facelift (but less than those in the normal weight range), as can those with flaws in bone structure, deep lines, thick folds, and heavy sagging. Expectations and attitude, as discussed earlier, are the most important qualifications.

Your Facelift Procedure

An SMAS facelift procedure takes two to four hours. Incision placement can vary. It's common for the surgeon to make an incision in the hairline from the temple to the ear, vertically in front of and behind the ear, and horizontally in the hairline, and another incision under the chin. Placement might be slightly different in men to prevent beard-growing skin from being reattached behind the ear. The operation involves several basic steps:

- The skin is separated from underlying fat and muscle.

- Some of the fat may be trimmed or suctioned.

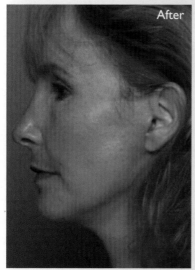

After

Facelift with eyelid lift and chin implant.

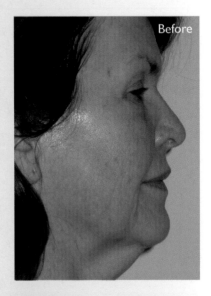

Before

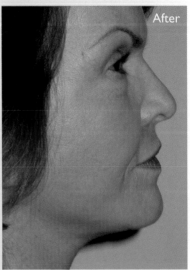

After

- Sometimes the SMAS is incised, lifted, and replaced so that the back edge overlaps the surrounding tissue; other times it is folded over itself. Lifting the SMAS brings the skin up and backward. The skin is redraped and the excess is trimmed.

- The skin is reattached. To prevent noticeable scarring, the redraped skin is not pulled tight and the incisions are closed without tension. Your doctor may use a combination of skin clips, removable sutures, and absorbable sutures.

After Your Facelift

You'll be given detailed postoperative instructions, similar to those outlined in Chapter 3. With instructions in hand, go home and relax! The first few days are critical for healing, though you'll need to be careful for several weeks. Any jarring of your face—by anything from a small child's sudden movement to a swinging door—could undo some of what your doctor so skillfully accomplished. Your doctor will likely emphasize that you should avoid bending over or lifting. When you do this, blood rushes to your head and can put pressure on delicate, healing tissues. You may be asked to avoid turning your head back and forth for the first few days.

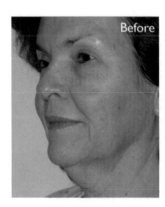

Before

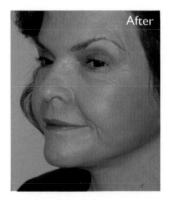

After

Facelift with modified deep chemical peel.

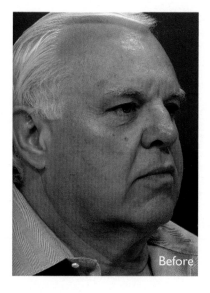

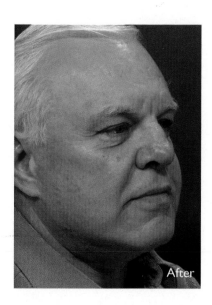

Before

After

Don't be surprised if your face feels numb, stiff, and a little sore at first. You'll also notice that your facial skin feels tight; this feeling will start to dissipate in a week or two. After a week or so you can probably return to work, depending on the type of work you do. Strenuous activity should be avoided for the first two weeks. Your doctor will give you detailed instructions for self-care at home.

Combining Facelifts with Other Procedures

Your facial plastic surgeon may suggest you have additional procedures before, after, or at the same time as your facelift. For example, many doctors routinely perform *liposuction*, using a suction tool to remove fat from under the skin, with a facelift. Similarly, your doctor may recommend lip augmentation, chin or cheek implants, a browlift, eyelid surgery, or nose reshaping. Facelifts won't eliminate all facial wrinkles or flaws in the skin, so if you wish to eliminate more wrinkles and improve the texture of your skin, you may wish to consider a chemical peel or laser skin resurfacing.

Questions to Ask Your Doctor

- After my surgery, should I use nonprescription products on my face to help the incisions heal? What products should I avoid?

- Can you give me a sample soft diet to follow after surgery? Should I avoid sodium to reduce swelling?

- How long will I need in-home assistance after surgery?

- I have heard that therapeutic massage can promote healing. Do you recommend this practice?

- How long will my facelift last?

- Will I need camouflage makeup and instructions to apply it?

CHAPTER 5

MIDFACE LIFT

MIDFACE LIFT

*N*o doubt you're quite familiar with what a facelift does. However, you might not be as familiar with a variation of the facelift known as a midface lift. This procedure is comparatively new to the facial cosmetic surgeon's repertoire, having been around only since the early 1990s. In fact, not every facial plastic surgeon performs a midface lift.

What Is a Midface Lift?

A *midface lift* restores the rounded facial contours with a surgical procedure that lifts and repositions the soft tissues between your eyes and mouth—the *midface*. The procedure improves hollows under your eyelids, raises your sagging cheeks, and smoothes your nasal furrows. The procedure is sometimes called a *cheek lift* or a *vertical lift* because in most cases surgeons pull the soft tissues almost straight up and reposition them above your cheekbones. Unlike a traditional facelift, a midface lift is usually done endoscopically, using a probe with a tiny camera and requiring very small incisions.

How long will a midface lift last? Of course, the results vary with each person; however, a midface lift should last five or six years. Lifestyle and skin care play a role in maintaining the results of a midface lift procedure.

Are You a Candidate?

Do you have sagging cheeks? Deep nasolabial folds? Do you have hollows or bags under your eyes or a scowling expression because the corners of your lips are downturned? If so, a midface lift might be an option for you. Men and women in their forties and older can enjoy the benefits of this procedure, as can people in their thirties who have hereditary midface flaws or early signs of aging.

A midface lift alone works best on people who wish to reverse signs of aging in the midface area.

The midface lift also works well as a follow-up procedure for those who have had previous lower facelifts. In fact, up to a third of midface lift patients are men or women who have already had facelifts but need another lift to the midface. Keep in mind that a midface lift does not remove sagging skin of the lower face or neck.

Your Midface Lift Procedure

Once you're fully sedated, your surgeon will lift at least the cheek fat pads to a position over the cheekbones and suspend them with sutures from a deeper structure, probably the muscles or deep tissues in your temple area. In a more extensive procedure, the buccal fat pad, those in the lower part of the face, and the fat pads under the eyes, known as the *suborbicularis oculi fat* (SOOF), are also repositioned. This variation on the procedure is often called a *SOOF lift.*

Incision placement depends on the technique being used. Incisions may be made on the inside or the outside of the lower eyelid. Or the doctor might make a series of small incisions above your hairline and possibly on the inside of your upper lip. Some midface lift procedures include small incisions above the ears. The operation will probably take 60 to 90 minutes.

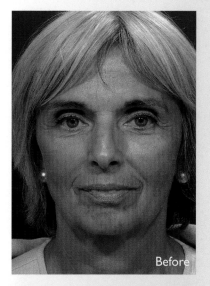

Before

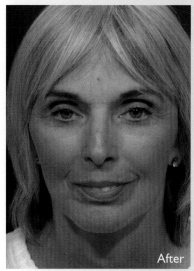

After

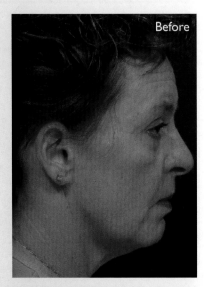

Before

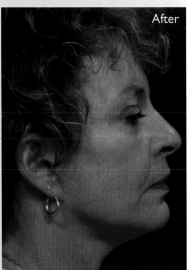

After

Surgeons also may perform midface lifts through incisions used in lower eyelid surgery. A less invasive method, *midface suspension,* involves lifting the cheek pads with suture loops attached at the temples.

Endoscopic Procedure

If your surgeon is performing the procedure endoscopically, it will be done with small incisions through which probes are inserted. On the inserted end of one probe is a miniature camera that projects images onto a monitor. Separating skin, muscle, and fat from bone and lifting the soft tissues are all performed through the small incisions.

With an endoscopic midface lift performed at the *subperiosteal* level, below the membrane covering the bone, the midface tissues are pulled up and anchored to the temporal muscles, which are in the temples. An endoscopic midface lift requires one to two hours.

After Your Midface Lift

You may be able to return to work anywhere from one to three weeks after surgery. By then most of the swelling will have subsided. When you can return to work will depend on your doctor's preference and the type and number of procedures you had. Your surgeon will give you specific self-care instructions.

Side Effects, Risks, and Complications

Expect temporary swelling, slight bruising, and numbness. If there's an incision in your mouth, you may feel it, but it is rarely uncomfortable. Rarely, with incisions in the lower eyelids, there can be some puckering at the corners of the eyes. This problem can be corrected in the doctor's office.

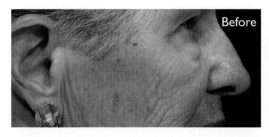

Before

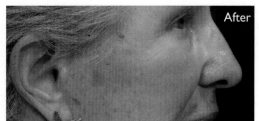

After

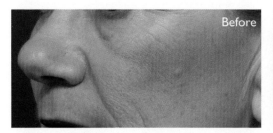

Before

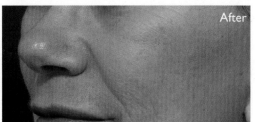

After

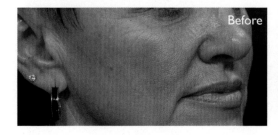

Before

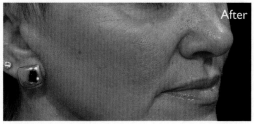

After

Questions to Ask Your Doctor

- Given my goals, is a midface lift best for me?

- How much downtime should I plan for?

- Can I still have a standard facelift later?

- How long will my midface lift last?

Combining Midface Lift with Other Procedures

You can have a midface lift alone or in combination with a facelift, eyelid surgery, cheek or tear-trough implants, browlifts, laser resurfacing, fat transfer, or Botox. Some procedures—chemical peels, for example—shouldn't be done at the same time as your midface lift. If you're having additional procedures, you and your doctor together will decide on the timing.

CHAPTER 6

EYELID LIFT

EYELID LIFT

*I*n classically beautiful eyes, you can see the entire pupil. Above it, some of the iris—the colored ring around the pupil—is visible. So is most of the iris below the pupil, but not the white of the eyeball, called the sclera. There is smooth skin between the upper lashes and the crease of the upper lid, and the eyes themselves are neither round nor narrow but somewhere in between, more almond-shaped.

If you look in the mirror and see white between the lower eyelid and the iris, or if you have developed dark circles or bags under the eyes, or drooping upper lids, eyelid surgery may be a procedure you'll wish to consider.

What Is Eyelid Surgery?

Eyelid surgery, or *blepharoplasty*—from blepharon, a Greek word meaning "eyelid," and *plasticos*, "to mold"—is surgery to rejuvenate the eyelids. The purpose of cosmetic eyelid surgery is to help restore your eyes' youthful beauty. As a bonus, the surgery might also help you see better if your upper lids are heavy and loose.

Why do your eyelids begin to droop? Your eyelids, thin as they seem, have several layers—skin, muscles, tendons, fat, connective tissue, and the *conjunctiva*, a thin, moist membrane that lines the underside of the eyelid and the exposed part of the eye. As we age, the eyelid skin becomes thinner and stretches. Also, the *orbicularis* muscles around the eyes weaken. Both skin and muscle begin to sag. The upper lids may drape over the lashes and, in some cases, restrict your vision. Often, fat around the eyes will *herniate* or protrude through weak places in the muscle and create bags under the eyes. If this occurs in the upper lids, they may look puffy.

How long will eyelid surgery last? Most patients find that they can enjoy the benefits of blepharoplasty for approximately ten years or longer. If one's brow begins to descend, it may appear that the results of eyelid surgery are fading, when in fact, the change is resulting from the shift in the brow.

Are You a Candidate?

Eyelid surgery can dramatically improve your appearance if your eyelids are puffy or drooping or if you have bags or hollows under your eyes. Generally, between the ages of thirty-five and forty is when people begin to notice these problems, though herniated fat in the lower eyelids can be an inherited trait that shows up in younger people. If you're in good health and you have realistic expectations from cosmetic surgery, you could be an excellent candidate.

Your doctor will want to make sure eyelid puffiness isn't a result of allergies or fluid and to rule out a medical cause of drooping eyelids. *Myxedema*, severe untreated hypothyroidism, can create the appearance of bulging eyes and fat around the eyes. Because thyroid disorders are common, especially in women over sixty, and since untreated thyroid problems can make you seriously ill, it's a good idea to have the simple blood test for thyroid function as part of your regular medical exam.

Your surgeon will examine your eyes and may also want an ophthalmologist to do so. If you have glaucoma, a detached retina, or dry-eye syndrome, your eyelid surgery may need to be postponed until these conditions are successfully treated.

If you have had eye surgery or facial paralysis, or if you have muscle laxness in your lower lid, cosmetic eyelid surgery might not be right for you.

Your Eyelid Surgery Procedure

On the morning of your surgery, clean your face thoroughly and don't apply any makeup. Be sure to take high-quality sunglasses to the hospital or surgical suite; you'll probably need to wear them home, even if it's dark outside.

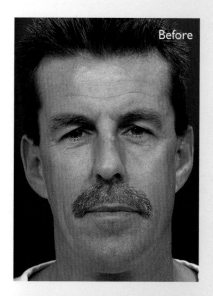

Before

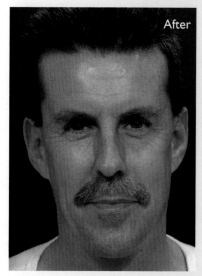

After

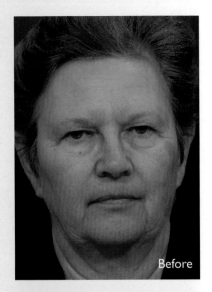

Before

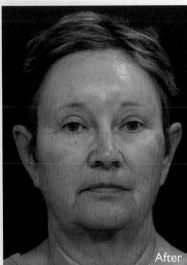

After

After eyelid lift, forehead lift, and midface lift.

Eyelid surgery is often an outpatient procedure. It can take as little as half an hour, though additional procedures will naturally require more time.

The doctor may recommend operating on both the upper and the lower eyelids. Eyelid surgery procedures differ according to where the incisions are placed and what is done with the excess tissue. Lower eyelid incisions may be *transcutaneous*—through the skin—or *transconjunctival*—on the underside of the eyelid, completely hidden. A transconjunctival approach has advantages. It prevents lower eyelid *retraction*, in which the lid becomes lax after surgery and may even pull away from the eye.

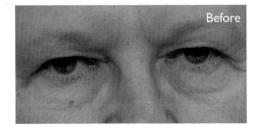
Before

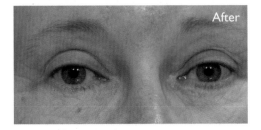
After

Sometimes skin and fat must be removed, and when the lower eyelid is already lax or there's a lot of extra skin, the lid must be tightened. In these cases, a transcutaneous incision is often a better choice. Though it's made through the skin, this incision is virtually invisible to others if it's done properly and it heals normally.

In some eyelid surgery procedures, fat is rearranged rather than removed. And although muscle, fat, and skin are all available for removal, the surgeon may remove (or reposition) only excess fat, especially in younger patients with herniated fat around the eyes but no skin sagging.

External incisions will be hidden in the natural creases of your eyelids. Upper lid tissues will be removed—fat, muscle, or skin, or a combination—and then the incisions will be closed. Your surgeon may use ordinary sutures or the type that dissolve on their own. If only fat is to be removed from your lower lids, the doctor will probably do so through incisions on the insides of the lids or with a laser. More extensive lower lid work—skin removal and lid tightening—may require transcutaneous (external) incisions. Sometimes doctors use a laser to sculpt upper lid fat that remains and to resurface lower lid skin. After closing the incisions, the surgeon may apply ointment to your eyes followed by cool compresses.

Many surgeons accomplish a similar result using lasers to remove lower eyelid fat bags, loose skin, and crows feet. With the patient sedated and the lid anesthetized, the surgeon turns down the lid and uses a CO_2 laser as a cutting tool to expose, remove, and sculpt the fat bags. The lid is then turned back, and the skin of the lower eyelid is resurfaced. This procedure removes 70 to 80 percent of the fine wrinkles and tightens the loose tissue.

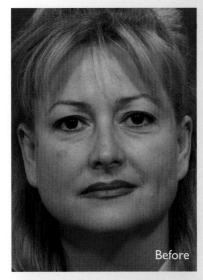

Before

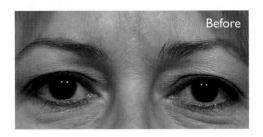

Before

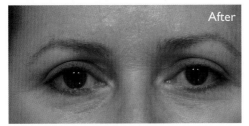

After

After Your Eyelid Surgery

In the recovery room, you'll probably experience nothing worse than some lid tightness or tenderness and perhaps blurred vision from the lubricating ointment. You'll lie with your head elevated and with cold compresses on your eyes to reduce swelling. When you're ready to go home, put on your sunglasses, even if it's dark or cloudy, for protection against airborne irritants.

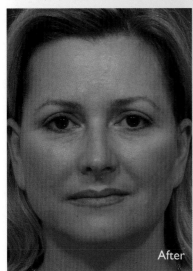

After

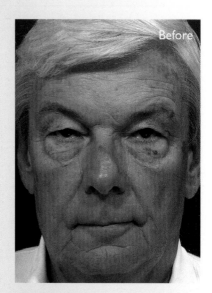

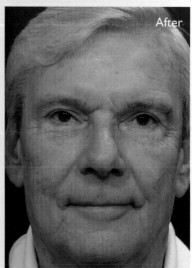

After upper and lower eyelid lift.

For the first few days, your doctor's orders will probably include frequent use of eye drops. You may be told not to do anything for long periods of time that might tire or dry out your eyes, such as reading, watching television, or using a computer. Avoid rubbing your eyes, and don't plan on wearing your contacts right away.

When you go out, wear sunglasses. Ultraviolet light can permanently darken scars. Your doctor might prescribe a sunscreen made just for eyelids.

Side Effects, Risks, and Complications

Call the doctor right away if you have severe pain, bulging eyes, or more than mild fluid buildup (edema); if your vision gets worse instead of better; or if numbness is more than very mild and short lived.

For the first week, your eyes may look bloodshot and you'll notice some swelling, slight bruising, and a "gumminess"—a change in the consistency of the protective tear film that covers your eyeball. This film is made up of water, oil, and mucus; after surgery, the composition of this film may change temporarily, so that it feels gummy rather than watery.

You might also experience tightness or difficulty closing your eyes; dry or watery eyes should last no more than a few days, but may persist for a few weeks. Blurred vision is often caused if the medicated ointment used on your incisions enters the eye; also, a temporary change in vision can result from the slight swelling around the eyeball. It is not unusual after eyelid surgery to develop tiny skin cysts, called *milia*, which may form on the scar line; these cysts may simply disappear or your doctor can remove them with a fine needle.

Head off potential problems by calling your doctor if an incision doesn't seem to be healing normally, a scar is getting darker rather than fading, or your eyes just don't seem to be working right after the first few days at home. Sometimes all that's needed is massage therapy or medication.

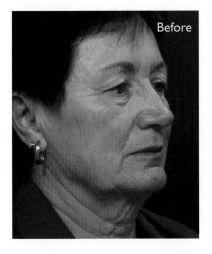
Before

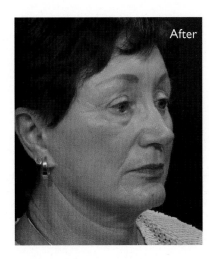
After

*Eyelid lift with
browlift and facelift.*

Combining Eyelid Surgery with Other Procedures

Sagging eyebrows may be causing some of the droopiness in your upper lids. If this is the case, talk to your doctor about having a *browlift*, also called a *forehead lift*, before or at the same time as eyelid surgery. If you do have a browlift, less skin will need to be removed from your eyelids. You might require an eyelid-tightening procedure if the lower lids are extremely lax. On the other hand, if laxity isn't severe, your surgeon may use a laser to tighten your lower lids rather than working through external incisions.

Some surgeons perform a midface lift with eyelid surgery, moving cheek tissue upward to fill grooves under the eyes. This can give much-needed support to the sagging lower eyelids and allow more to be done to improve the lower eyelid "aged look." If the skin under your eyes is darkly pigmented, bleaching or a chemical peel may help. Botox injections, chemical peels, and laser resurfacing might also improve your eyelid surgery results by softening laugh lines at the outside corners of your eyes. Before your eyelid surgery, your doctor will discuss the advantages and the optimal timing of additional procedures.

Questions to Ask the Surgeon

- Will the surgery affect my vision?

- Do I need to follow a special diet after surgery?

- How long will the results last? Will I need additional surgery down the road?

- What's the best type of cold compress to use during recovery? Do you recommend a special mask for sleeping?

- What vitamins and other supplements, if any, can I safely take before and after surgery?

CHAPTER 7

BROWLIFT

BROWLIFT

*T*he aging that can affect the face, neck, and eyelids can also affect our brows. As tissues of the brow weaken and the skin becomes thinner, we will see changes in the brow. It can start to slide downward. If your eyebrows or upper lids look and feel heavy, the brow is partially responsible much of the time.

Since forehead lines and sagging brows are among the earliest visible signs of aging, browlifts are a common cosmetic procedure men and women seek to regain their younger, warmer, more welcoming appearance.

What Is a Browlift?

If your eyebrow is low, look in the mirror and lift it gently with your fingers, observing the effect it has on brightening the eye. This is what a browlift accomplishes. Several procedures, collectively known as browlifts or forehead lifts, can rejuvenate the look of your forehead, eyes, and eyebrows. These procedures may elevate your brows, eliminate lines in the forehead, and correct heavy upper eyelids by removing, tightening, or repositioning tissues, including skin, muscle, and fat. A browlift can also reshape your eyebrows, giving them an attractive arch where they might otherwise be flat. Since a browlift gives the eyes a more open look, it allows women to once again apply makeup to the skin under their eyebrows.

Sometimes, overactive muscles in the forehead are responsible for a furrowed or heavy-lidded look. These muscles include the *procerus*, which wrinkles the upper nose; the *corrugator*, which causes frown lines to appear between the eyebrows; and the *frontalis*, which raises the eyebrows. Browlift surgery can remove, tighten, clip, or realign these muscles, diminishing the wrinkles they create.

A browlift can last from five to ten years, depending on lifestyle factors and maintained health.

Types of Browlifts

Browlifts are classified primarily by incision type and location. Your surgeon will advise you on the type of browlift most likely to achieve your goals.

Endoscopic (Minimal-Incision)

The *endoscopic* or *minimal-incision* browlift is the most commonly used technique for browlifts. The procedure is performed through three to five small incisions, usually a half-inch to an inch long. To guide the surgical instruments, the doctor inserts a miniature camera, which projects in ~~~~ onto a television monitor. Rather than being removed, excess skin is typically repositioned.

The surgeon lifts the forehead tissues upward and outward to give the brow the desired look. Once these tissues are healed, they will stay firmly in place. However, until healing occurs, they need to be "anchored." This is accomplished in a variety of ways. Some facial plastic surgeons create bone tunnels to anchor the tissue with a stitch. Others use small titanium screws in the bone or small absorbable plates. These plates are the size and thickness of a dime and have small spikes that hold the brow tissue like Velcro. After some months, they disappear as the body absorbs them.

The endoscopic approach has several advantages, including smaller incisions, nearly invisible scars, less swelling, and faster recovery.

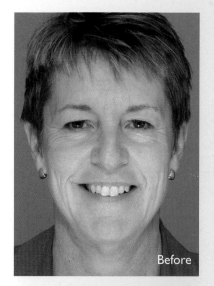
Before

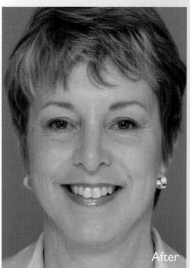
After

Browlift combined with facelift.

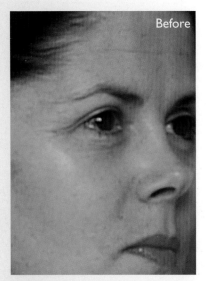

Before

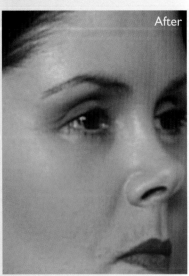

After

Coronal

Once considered standard, the *coronal* browlift is being used less often than it once was. It involves an incision that goes from ear to ear across the top of the head. The surgeon may remove up to an inch of the scalp, raising the brow. This is definitely not the recommended procedure for men who have receding hairlines or who are balding, or for anyone with a high forehead, since it tends to raise the hairline even further.

Pretrichial or Trichophytic

If you have a high forehead, your surgeon might prefer using a *pretrichial* (or *anterior hairline*) incision, which is just in front of the hairline. An advantage to this procedure is that a high hairline can be lowered. The surgeon has another option—a *trichophytic* incision, which is made a few millimeters inside the hairline using beveled incision through which the hair can regrow. This technique can preserve or in some cases lower the hairline, but there is a risk of visible scarring and permanent numbness.

Midforehead

Sometimes, in male patients especially, the surgeon may place the incision in one of the forehead's deep horizontal furrows. Although this type of procedure is not used as frequently as other approaches, it may work well for a bald man, who is not able to conceal incision scars on top of the head.

Temporal

In this procedure, small diamond-shape *temporal* incisions are made at the hairline on either side of the forehead. This procedure, also called a *lateral* browlift, may not be as extensive as a coronal or pretrichial incision, but scars can be well hidden in most patients. There is a lower risk of numbness. Improvement might not last as long as with other approaches.

Direct

The *direct browlift* may be used in men whose eyebrows are heavy enough to hide scars. This is a relatively simple procedure in which skin just above the eyebrows is removed. This is rarely done because scars are almost certainly visible to some extent, and because the procedure may feminize the male brow by giving it a more "straight across" look, which resembles a plucked brow.

Are You a Candidate?

Browlift candidates can be any age, though most are between forty and seventy. Some people are born with a hereditary low browline, which can become unattractive once the skin is no longer taut and smooth. These people may decide to have browlift surgery early, even in their thirties.

What signs should you look for if you're considering a browlift? The procedure can improve a sagging forehead, which often contributes to sagging upper eyelids, low brows too close to the eyes, frown lines or deep forehead furrows, and a weary, sad, or angry appearance. Don't rule out a browlift if you're bald, you have a high forehead, or you've already had eyelid surgery. There are many approaches your doctor can choose from, some more conservative than others, but still effective.

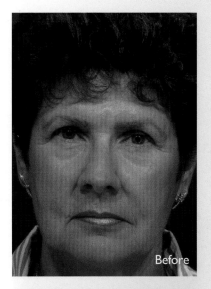

Before

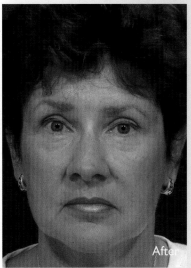

After

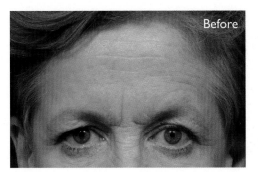

Before

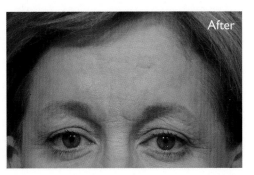

After

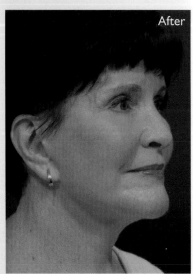

Before

After

Browlift combined with facelift.

Your Browlift Procedure

Before the procedure, your hair will be gathered into sections with clips or rubber bands. Occasionally the part of the hair around the incision is clipped or shaved, though this is usually unnecessary.

A browlift alone takes as little as 30 minutes. After making the incisions according to the type of browlift chosen, the surgeon will lift all the tissues together off the bone and move them upward and outward. They'll be secured (or fixed) in the new position until they heal.

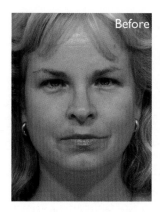
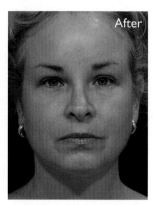

Before

After

Several methods of fixation are available to the surgeon. One is a small absorbable plate attached to the bone; this plate disappears after several months as the body digests it. No drains are needed. In other cases, your doctor may reattach tissues with sutures, skin clips, or tissue glue. Platelet gel is also used.

After the incisions are closed, a dressing or elastic band might be wrapped around your head to keep the repositioned tissues and gauze pads in place and to reduce swelling. If your doctor has used tissue glue or platelet-rich plasma, there will probably be no drains or external dressings.

After Your Browlift

Recovering at home involves following your doctor's instructions and taking it easy for several days. During your first follow-up appointment, the surgeon will remove your bandages and drains, if any, and examine your incisions.

Side Effects, Risks, and Complications

Your forehead, cheeks, and the skin around your eyes may be swollen. Because sensory nerves may have been disturbed during surgery, you may experience areas of numbness. Your healing timeline will vary—shorter if your surgery was endoscopic, longer if you had a coronal or pretrichial incision.

At first, your brow might look asymmetrical. One eyebrow might be higher than the other, or both might appear too high. As healing progresses, the look will even out and you'll begin to see your new, smoother contours.

Combining Browlifts with Other Procedures

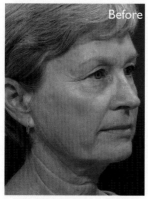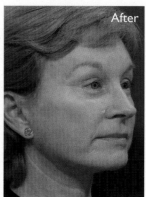

Browlift combined with facelift.

If you are in your thirties or early forties, a browlift alone might very well give you the younger, fresher, friendlier look you're hoping for. Older patients who want facial rejuvenation, however, will probably not be satisfied with a browlift alone, even if sagging brows are the most obvious sign of aging.

Browlifts are often performed with facelifts, midface lifts, eyelid lifts, or other procedures—at the same time or separated by several weeks. Many surgeons routinely do Botox treatments or laser eyelid resurfacing in conjunction with forehead lifts. Sometimes upper eyelids can be corrected and frown lines removed through the same incisions. There are many possible combinations, and your doctor can use computer imaging to give you an idea of what results you can expect with one or more procedures.

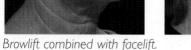

Questions to Ask Your Doctor

- Will a browlift give me the look I want, or do I need eyelid surgery as well?

- Am I a candidate for an endoscopic procedure?

- How long will the results of my browlift last?

- Do I need to protect my incision lines with sunblock?

- How long should I stay indoors after surgery?

- Is massage useful in healing scars and tissues? Can I learn the techniques myself?

CHAPTER 8

RHINOPLASTY

RHINOPLASTY

*N*oses are noticed, particularly if they are unusual. The large or crooked nose draws attention. And in our culture, whether we find it appropriate or not, someone's nose can affect how we perceive him or her. The nose often symbolizes intelligence, masculinity or femininity, even strength of character. A nose that's in harmony with other features gives the face a pleasing balance.

It comes as no surprise then that rhinoplasty, the medical term for a "nose job," is the most common facial cosmetic procedure performed in the United States. More than 350,000 Americans have this procedure every year. About 60 percent of rhinoplasty patients are women.

What Is Rhinoplasty?

Nasal refinement, or *rhinoplasty*, is surgery to reshape the nose. The procedure can make your nose straighter, wider or narrower, longer or shorter. It can change the shape of the tip or bridge. It can change the angle between the nose and upper lip or narrow the nostrils. *Tiplasty* may be performed when only the tip of the nose needs refinement. Shortening the nose, often by lifting the tip, can make you look younger.

Although nose reshaping is a cosmetic procedure, the procedure can also correct an existing breathing problem. For example, during rhinoplasty a surgeon can repair a deviated (crooked) septum, which may block the airflow on one side of the nose. The septum is the wall of bone and cartilage that separates the nostrils. This operation is called *septoplasty*.

Rhinoplasty is considered a permanent procedure; certainly bone and cartilage removed will not grow back. However, as we age our noses do become a bit longer as ligaments and other tissue lose some of their tension.

Types of Rhinoplasty

Each procedure is tailored to the needs of the individual patient; however, there are two basic types of rhinoplasty. The first is *open rhinoplasty*, which involves placing a small incision across the *columella*, the strip of tissue separating the nostrils, along with incisions inside the nose. The second type is *closed rhinoplasty*, in which only internal incisions are used. Most facial plastic surgeons agree that the best approach is the one the doctor prefers. Open rhinoplasty is sometimes necessary for unusually complex procedures and revision procedures.

Are You a Candidate?

If you've been self-conscious about your nose for as long as you can remember, rhinoplasty can help you find new self-assurance. For all patients, the goal is balanced and attractive facial contours, not an ideal nose. If you're an adult in good emotional and physical health, and you want improvement rather than perfection, you could be an excellent candidate for cosmetic surgery of the nose.

Teenagers can have the procedure after they have finished their growth spurt, usually by age fifteen or sixteen. If you're in your teens, your doctor will want to be sure you're seeking the surgery because you want it and not because you're doing it out of parental or peer pressure.

Ethnicity is a factor in some rhinoplasty procedures. You and your doctor can best decide how much to soften a bump, for example, or narrow the base of the nose and still achieve harmony with the rest of your features—focusing on *your face* and its individual, distinctive attractiveness.

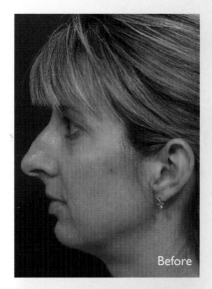

Before

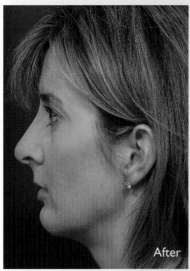

After

Rhinoplasty combined with chin implant, which achieves better facial balance.

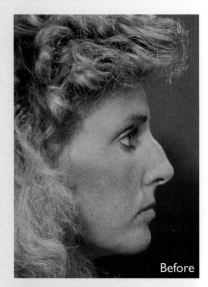

Before

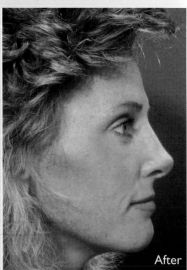

After

Many people seek rhinoplasty after a nasal fracture. Your surgeon will want to wait several months after the injury, until the swelling goes down, before performing the procedure.

Any injury to your nose, respiratory conditions (such as asthma) that cause breathing problems, and smoking or recreational drug use can affect the method and timing of your rhinoplasty. Avoid irritating your nose in any way before the operation; if it is sunburned, puffy, or inflamed, surgery may need to be postponed.

If you're unhappy with an earlier rhinoplasty, you may be a candidate for *revision rhinoplasty* a year or more after the first procedure, which must heal completely before new surgery is performed.

Your Rhinoplasty Procedure

The operation usually takes one to three hours. Once you're sedated, small incisions will be made. Through these incisions, the doctor will separate the skin from the underlying bone and cartilage. External incisions, virtually invisible once healed, are hidden in the creases of the nose.

Depending on the structure of your nose and the desired result, your surgeon may use one or more of these techniques:

- Narrow or widen the bridge
- Maneuver bone and cartilage to sculpt the new shape
- File or chisel excess bone at the hump
- Remove small wedges of skin to narrow the base of the nose
- Suture to narrow flared nostrils
- Trim cartilage at the tip
- Add nasal cartilage, or bone or cartilage from another part of your body, to build up the nose.

Once the nose is reshaped, the doctor will then redrape the skin and soft tissues over the new structure. He or she will probably apply an external splint and may place soft rubber or plastic splints or absorbent material inside the nose. These protect the nose from bumps, maintain the new shape, and keep the nasal structures in place during the early part of healing. Finally, the surgeon will put a gauze drip pad under your nose to absorb blood and mucus.

It used to be common practice for doctors to pack the nose with long strips of Vaseline-coated gauze. This was done to support the nose and prevent bleeding. However, it is usually uncomfortable for patients when it's time to remove the packing from the tender, healing nose. As a result, today there is a trend toward doctors not packing the nose, but rather using special suturing to support the nose and prevent bleeding.

After Your Rhinoplasty

You'll probably go home the same day of your surgery. Most doctors will want to see you the next day. If your nose was packed with gauze, it will probably be removed the first or second day after your surgery. Your doctor will likely instruct you to sleep only on your back with your head elevated for the first week after your surgery. You will be able to return to work or school in as little as three days.

You'll visit the doctor again within a week for another follow-up appointment. At that time, splints will be gently removed. Sutures, if not the absorbable kind, may be removed. Take your eyeglasses to the visit. Some doctors advise taping your glasses to your forehead for several weeks or supporting them another way until the nose is healed.

You'll see a change in your nose immediately after surgery; however, complete healing can take six months to a year. It often takes this long for all the swelling to subside. In some cases, your friends and family may say they can't see any difference.

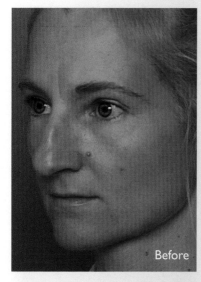

Before

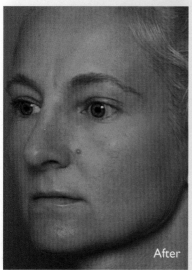

After

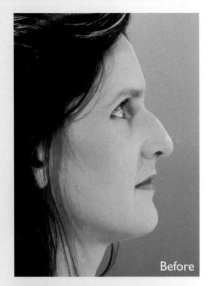

Before

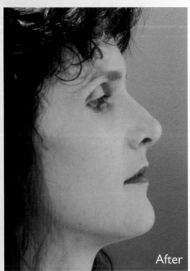

After

Improvement can be subtle and gradual, but if you've chosen a first-rate surgeon, there will be improvement that you'll be aware of even if others are not.

Cleaning the Skin on Your Nose

Until the splint is removed, about a week after surgery, you won't be able to clean your nose, inside or out. After the doctor removes the splint, you can gently clean the skin on your nose with a mild, nonabrasive cleanser or soap. Use cotton or a soft sponge, not a terry washcloth, and don't scrub. Your doctor may suggest carefully cleaning the incision area just inside the nose with petroleum jelly on a clean Q-tip (not on your fingers), and using hydrogen peroxide on a Q-tip to clean the external incision.

Avoid Sneezing

When you feel a sneeze coming on, sneeze through your mouth, not your nose. Sneezing may disturb the healing soft tissues inside your nose. Sneezing is common after rhinoplasty, and your doctor may prescribe an antihistamine to keep it to a minimum. Also, avoid blowing your nose though it may feel congested for several weeks.

Side Effects

You'll have clear mucous drainage for the first few days, with some blood the first night. Occasionally, there is a small amount of blood in the drainage for a few days. Change the gauze pad as often as needed. Rarely, a patient will have a runny nose for several months.

The inside of your nose may be swollen and the incisions may be crusty for several weeks; this may affect breathing through your nose. Breathing through your mouth is drying, so keep water and lip lubricants handy. You might want to sleep with a humidifier running.

Some patients swallow blood during surgery; this may cause short-term nausea and dark stools. If you rest and take in only clear liquids, the nausea should be gone in a day or so. Tell your doctor if your stomach continues to be upset or if you are vomiting.

You may have a low-grade fever and chills for a day or two. Call the doctor if your temperature is more than two degrees above what's normal for you.

Risks and Complications

Nosebleeds are unusual after rhinoplasty, occurring in fewer than one percent of patients. Don't worry if you do get a nosebleed. Simply lie back (not completely flat) with your head elevated and place a soft ice bag or an ice-cold washcloth over your nose. Until the nose stops bleeding, don't bend over or do anything else that might raise your blood pressure. Relaxing is essential to allow the bleeding to stop.

In very few patients, small burst blood vessels appear on the skin as tiny red dots. These may eventually disappear and in any case are inconspicuous.

Other rare complications include nerve injury, injury to the septum, obstruction of nasal passages, permanent numbness, allergic reaction to sutures, and toxic shock syndrome. If a skilled, experienced surgeon performs your procedure, the risk of serious complications is much less than one percent.

Combining Rhinoplasty with Other Procedures

It's not uncommon for facial plastic surgeons to recommend *chin augmentation* along with rhinoplasty, since a small chin can make the nose look larger. In fact, chin augmentation is usually recommended in about 10 percent of rhinoplasty patients. You might also benefit from laser skin resurfacing or eyelid surgery at the time of your nose reshaping. More complex procedures, such as facelifts, may be done a week or more before or after rhinoplasty, or at the same time.

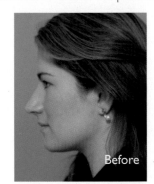
Before

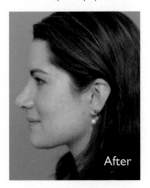
After

Questions to Ask the Surgeon

- Will I have nasal packing after surgery?

- Can I use concealing makeup to cover bruising?

- When will I see what my new nose looks like?

- When can I go back to work?

CHAPTER 9

OTOPLASTY

OTOPLASTY

*A*re you self-conscious about your ears? Do they protrude or are they slightly deformed? If so, you have a condition that can be treated with an operation known as **otoplasty**. The procedure can make your ears smaller or bring them closer to your head, giving them natural curves and contours.

Sometimes referred to as "pinning back" the ears, the procedure is considered safe and effective, and in recent years it has become an increasingly popular procedure.

What Is Otoplasty?

Otoplasty is cosmetic surgery to the *auricle*—the outer portion of the ear—usually done to correct protruding ears, the most common complaint of otoplasty patients. Plastic surgeons can also address a range of deformities caused by genetics or injury and can even construct and attach new ears. The procedure has no effect on the inner ear, so you don't need to worry about your hearing being damaged while your ears are being beautified.

The visible part of the ear—the *auricle*—consists of cartilage, connective tissue, and skin. When an ear protrudes, a section of cartilage may be missing or overdeveloped. Less common ear irregularities can range from *asymmetry*—when one ear looks markedly different from the other—to a misshapen "cauliflower ear" caused by injury. Other ear abnormalities include:

- *Constricted ear:* The outer rim is tightened, hooded, or folded.

- *Cup ear:* A type of constricted ear in which the part of the ear folds down, part of it is enlarged, and the ear protrudes. This combination of factors makes the ear look unusually small.

- *Lobes* that are enlarged, stretched, or creased.

- *Lop ear:* Another type of constricted ear in which the top is folded down and forward and the "scooped out" section of the ear is at a right angle to the head. Sometimes called *bat ear*.

- *Macrotia:* The ear is too big. True macrotia is rare; protrusion is the usual cause of ears appearing too big.

- *Microtia:* The ear is too small.

- *Shell ear:* The fold of the helix and other natural folds and creases are missing.

- *Stahl's ear:* The helix is flattened and the auricle's upper edge is pointed. There may be an extra fold, or the scapha may be bent forward. Sometimes called *Spock's ear* or *Vulcan ear*.

- *Telephone ear:* The top and bottom of the auricle stick out farther than the rest of the ear.

Types of Otoplasty

Otoplasty may be *cartilage sparing* or *cartilage splitting*. Cartilage-sparing techniques may include sculpting cartilage by filing or bending and suturing. Cartilage splitting involves cutting the cartilage; this approach may create angles that disturb the smooth contours of the auricle, especially in adults, if not done well. This surgery produces permanent results.

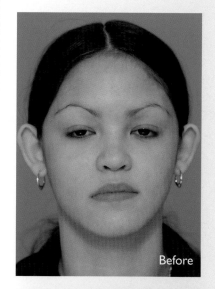
Before

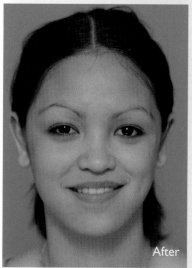
After

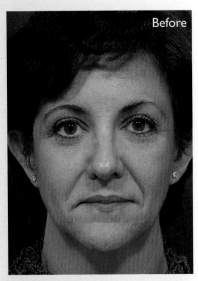

Before

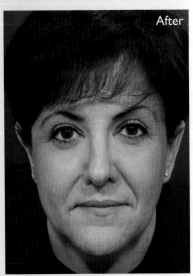

After

Are You a Candidate?

Adults who are self-conscious about their ears and who are in good physical and emotional health are usually excellent candidates for otoplasty. Though their ear cartilage is more rigid than that of children, the surgery is safe and effective.

Your Otoplasty Procedure

Your surgeon may perform the operation in an accredited in-office surgical suite or an outpatient surgery center. Some doctors prefer to do the procedure in a hospital with an overnight stay, especially if the patient is a child or if general anesthesia is used. Ask your doctor about the hospital's arrangements for parents who wish to stay overnight with their children.

Though some otoplasty procedures can be done in as little as an hour, most surgeons estimate two hours for the operation. Young children usually sleep through the operation under general anesthesia. Older children and adults will likely have a local anesthetic combined with an IV sedative and will be able to go home the same day.

Even if only one ear is affected, cosmetic surgeons usually operate on both ears for a balanced, symmetrical result. Working through a small, football-shaped incision in the back of the ear, the surgeon may fold cartilage, holding it in position with permanent sutures; the surgeon may also remove excess cartilage or add cartilage to rebuild folds. Other techniques may also be used, depending on the revision being made. Sometimes the desired results can be obtained with sutures within the ear cartilage or to the deep tissues of the scalp.

Your ears aren't like anyone else's, so no two otoplasty procedures are alike. Your doctor may sculpt your new ear with any of the following techniques:

- Trimming, shaving, flattening, or folding cartilage and bending it back toward the head.

- Pinning the cartilage closer to the head with permanent sutures (which will not be visible to you or anyone else after surgery).

- Removing a sliver of cartilage and reattaching the edges with sutures.

- Removing skin, but not cartilage, using permanent sutures to reshape the ear.

- Trimming tissue from elongated earlobes.

The surgeon will then redrape the skin over the newly sculpted ear and close the incision with dissolvable or removable sutures (or both). Multiple layers of sutures will help the ear keep its new shape while it is healing.

Bandages will be applied to protect the ears and maintain their shape. Your doctor may saturate cotton with antibiotic ointment, mold it in the crevices of the ears, and cover it with thick padding, which will be removed in one to three days. Meanwhile, you'll probably be told not to touch the bandages.

After Your Otoplasty

Your ears will be bandaged for a few days, but once the bandages are off, you'll see improvement immediately. Though the cartilage of adults' ears is not as pliable as that of children, otoplasty patients of all ages are usually delighted with their more attractive, better proportioned ears.

During the first week after surgery your doctor will probably remove bandages and sutures and instruct you to wear a wide elastic headband throughout the day for one to three weeks and at night for up to six weeks. The headband will help keep your newly sculpted ears in place and allow them to heal in the proper position. You should keep your head above your heart—don't bend over—for about three more weeks.

For as long as your bandages are in place, keep them dry. Ask the doctor for instructions about showering and washing your hair. If you use a hair dryer, keep it

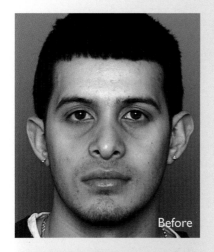

Before

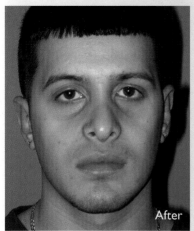

After

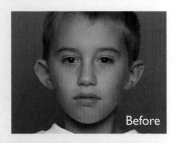

Before

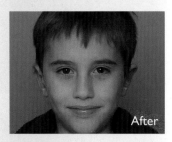

After

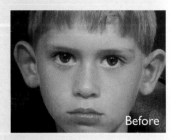

Before

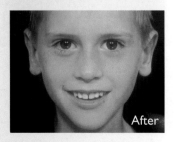

After

on the low setting, and don't use a curling iron, electric rollers, or anything else that might overheat or burn your ears, which might be a bit numb and insensitive to the burning sensation.

For about a month, sleep on your back, not your stomach or your side. Pressure on the ear can interfere with correct healing.

Side Effects

When the bandages first come off, your once-protruding ears may look *hypercorrected*—too close to the head—though you'll notice improvement right away. As your ears heal, they'll settle into their permanent positions.

Though most patients feel fine after otoplasty, the bulky bandages can be uncomfortably hot and the healing process may make your ears itch. Do not give into the urge to scratch them; if the itching persists, you may wish to call your doctor, who may prescribe an oral or topical medication to reduce the itching.

Risks and Complications

Thousands of otoplasty procedures are performed each year, on children and adults alike, with no ill effects. Rare complications can usually be handled with medication or minor surgery. You can almost always reduce the risks yourself by choosing an experienced, reputable surgeon and by faithfully following his or her instructions before and after the operation. Though extremely unlikely, complications can occur.

- *Suture bridging.* Permanent sutures can be seen through the skin; this is a result of too much skin being removed during the procedure.

- *Chondritis.* Infection in the cartilage, which can create scar tissue. Infections can typically be managed with antibiotics and rarely need to be drained.

- *Unsatisfactory results,* including asymmetry, undercorrection, overcorrection, or an unnatural appearance of the ear.

- *Loss of correction.* Recurrence of the protrusion or other defect may occur if the sutures loosen or break, either because the doctor has placed the sutures improperly or the patient hasn't adequately protected the ears after surgery.

Otoplasty for Children

More than half of otoplasty patients are under eighteen years old, and most of these young patients are between four and fourteen. There are two schools of thought about when children should have otoplasty. Some professionals feel strongly that children as young as four, and no older than five or six, should have the procedure before socialization takes root, the teasing becomes too hurtful, and the victims develop psychological scars. Besides, the younger the child, the softer and more pliable the cartilage. According to these physicians and counselors, the parents in consultation with a plastic surgeon should make the decision. No child, however, should be dragged kicking and screaming into surgery.

The other school of thought argues that surgery should wait until children are unhappy about their appearance and want the procedure. Children eight and older can understand and follow their doctors' instructions, before and after surgery, better than younger children.

In any case, surgical correction for children must wait until their ears are nearly finished growing, usually between the ages of four and six. The child should have a positive attitude, and the parents' primary concern must be the child's well being and not any embarrassment they might feel about their child's appearance.

Children can usually go back to school after a week of rest and quiet activity. If your child is overly active during that first week, talk to the doctor. Once children are back at school, they should stay off the playground and out of gym class until the doctor permits.

Questions to Ask Your Doctor

- How long will I need to wear a bandage?

- How soon after surgery can I take a shower or wash my hair?

- What are the most important things I can do to prevent complications?

- Are the results permanent?

CHAPTER 10

WRINKLE FILLERS

10

WRINKLE FILLERS

acial cosmetic surgery can produce dramatic results. A facelift can turn back the clock many years. Even so, we can still be left with fine lines, folds, or wrinkles that aren't always eliminated with a facelift. It is standard practice today for facial cosmetic surgeons to use other procedures to complement the surgery. Soft-tissue fillers, often referred to as "wrinkle fillers," fill in wrinkles and grooves or creases, blending them into the rest of your skin.

What Are Fillers?

Fillers are the materials used to plump up wrinkles or folds in the skin. They come in two forms: injections and implants. Filler injections are typically used for nasolabial folds, forehead lines, crow's feet, smile lines, frown lines, and the fine wrinkles around the lips. Filler implant material is frequently used to fill creases in the cheeks, to improve wrinkled lips, or to fill in nasolabial folds. Fillers may be either temporary or permanent.

Types of Temporary Fillers

Fillers are considered temporary when the material used is eventually reabsorbed by the body. Temporary fillers can also provide an ideal way to try out a wrinkle-filling or tissue-lifting technique before considering a more permanent method. Fillers are popular because they are quick and involve virtually no downtime. They are delivered by injection.

Collagen

Collagen injections are effective for the correction of fine smile or frown lines, nasolabial folds, delicate lines at the corners of the eyes or around the lips, and acne scars. Collagen is a natural protein, a substance that forms part of the supporting structure under the skin. However, our own supplies of collagen naturally diminish with age. Using collagen for cosmetic purposes was first introduced in the United States nearly twenty years ago. During that time, most collagen fillers were derived from purified bovine (cow) collagen.

In March 2003, the FDA approved the first human-source collagen products, made from purified human collagen under controlled laboratory conditions. Marketed as CosmoDerm™ and CosmoPlast,™ these products are expected to gain popularity because they eliminate the concern over allergic reactions to bovine collagen.

Both forms of collagen are temporary fillers. The treatments last from three to six months.

Hyaluronic Acid

Our bodies produce *hyaluronic acid,* a structural part of the skin that creates volume and shape and acts as a lubricant and shock absorber, but our natural supplies diminish with age. Synthetic gels, marketed under the names Restylane,™ Perlane,™ and Hylaform™ are very similar to natural hyaluronic acid. (Restylane and Perlane are the same product; Perlane is more highly concentrated.)

How do they work? The substance stimulates one's own natural skin cells to float upward to the surface of the skin. As a result, creases and grooves are filled in more naturally. This makes these injections particularly useful for treating nasolabial folds, lip lines, smile lines, and drooping corners of the mouth. They are also used to fill fine to moderate wrinkles as well as scars. The results last for about six to twelve months.

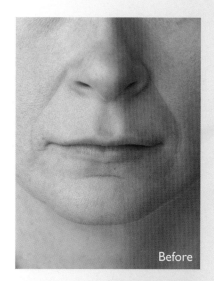

Before

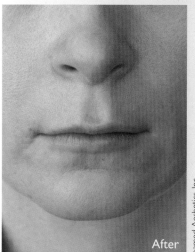

After

Inamed Aesthetics, Inc.

Collagen injections are used here to soften nasolabial folds.

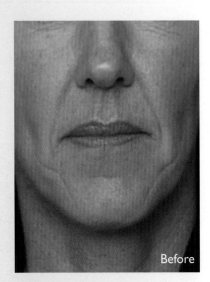
Before

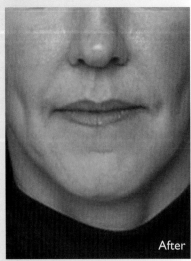
After

Two strands of implant material are threaded under the skin to soften the nasolabial folds.

Autologous Fat

Injections of your own autologous body fat can be used to reduce deeper facial wrinkles or fill in the hollows that have gradually appeared. These fat deposits can be drawn from the buttocks, thighs, or abdomen and are quickly processed into injectable form in the doctor's office. Sometimes the fat is extracted during a mini-liposuction procedure or taken from a simple incision in an area such as the back of the knee. Because this is your body's own tissue, there is no risk of allergy or rejection.

In some people, the results last only a month or two; in others, they last years. Note that sometimes the area injected with the fat may become lumpy as the fat is reabsorbed by the body.

Fascia

Another treatment derived from your own or donor tissue, this filler consists of tiny pieces of the *fascia*, the firm, white collagen-rich layer that covers the muscles, just underneath body fat. Fascia is commonly harvested from the muscle above the ear through a small incision above the hairline. Originally small pieces were used only in surgery to fill deep scars, but it is now possible to process fascia into an injectable substance used to augment lips and smooth wrinkles. Like autologous fat, fascia lata is sometimes used as an alternative for people who show an allergic response to bovine collagen. Results should last three to six months.

Temporary Injectables						
	Hyaluronic acid	**Botulinum toxin**	**Fat injections**	**Hydroxylopatite**	**Collagen**	
Trade name	Restylane, Perlane, Restylane Fine Lines, Hylaform	Botox, Myobloc	Fat Injection	Radiesse	Zyderm, Zyplast	CosmoDerm, CosmoPlast
What it is	A substance found in all living organisms	Botulinum toxin type A, produced by *Clostridia Botulinum bacteria*	Fat transfer from one part of the body to another	Similar to a substance found in our bodies	Natural substances derived from purified bovine (cow) collagen	Human collagen developed in a laboratory
How it works	For volume and shaping	Temporarily relaxes the muscle	Adds volume	Adds volume	Adds volume	Adds volume
Injection areas	Nasolabial folds, forehead wrinkles, smile lines, lips	Forehead, frown lines, crow's feet, vertical neck bands	Nasolabial folds, frown lines, crow's feet, lips, facial recontouring	Nasolabial folds, marionette lines, lips	Nasolabial folds, frown lines, crow's feet, lips	Nasolabial folds, frown lines, crow's feet, lips
Results	Up to 12 months	Up to 6 months	Highly variable, months to years	2 to 5 years	Up to 6 months	Up to 6 months
U.S. availability	Yes	Yes	Yes	Yes	Yes	Yes
Back to work	No downtime	No downtime	7–14 days	1–2 days	No downtime	No downtime
Possible reactions	Swelling, redness, tenderness	Bruising, redness, droopy eyelid, headache, flu-like symptoms	Swelling, bruising, lumpiness	Swelling, bruising, lumpiness	Slight bruising, allergic reactions	Slight bruising, allergic reactions
Other considerations	None identified at this time	None identified at this time	Requires a donor site (for example, abdomen, buttocks, or thighs)	None at this time	Requires a skin test for allergic reaction and at least one-month wait	No pretreatment skin test required

Courtesy American Society for Aesthetic Plastic Surgery.

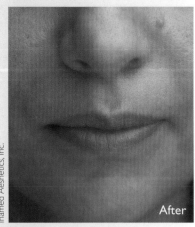

Before

After

Softening of nasolabial folds with hyaluronic acid.

Types of Permanent Fillers

Permanent fillers can give results ranging from semipermanent to permanent. Some of the newer permanent fillers are liquid blends of natural materials and tiny particles of vinyl or polymer. Other permanent fillers are solid or mesh-like implants, inserted through tiny incisions.

Hybrids

One of the newer filler products, known as a hybrid filler, is considered permanent. Marketed under the brand name Artefil™, it is a blend of microscopic plastic beads and human collagen. The body absorbs the collagen in a few months, but the permanent tiny beads stimulate the production of the body's own collagen. The new collagen encapsulates the beads, making the filler permanent.

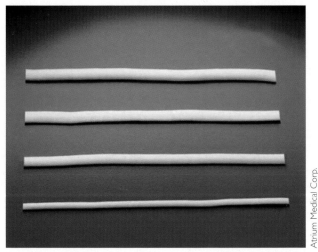

Samples of synthetic fillers. These strips of Advanta implant material are used to fill nasolabial folds and to augment lips.

The result: skin volume is boosted. The hybrid filler may be used for wrinkles, deep nasolabial folds, frown lines, and acne scars. Although used by some physicians, Artefil has not yet received official FDA approval.

Synthetic Implants

These solid, permanent implants are made from a medical-grade polymer similar to Gore-Tex™, the rubber used to make boots and raincoats. The polymer is firm but flexible. The implants come in various forms and shapes, including sheets, mesh-like strips, oval pieces, and round, tubular threads. Synthetic implants are often used for filling nasolabial folds.

Silicone

One well-known though controversial permanent filler treatment is silicone. Liquid silicone has been offered for years in microdroplet injection form by some physicians who believe that, used appropriately, it is safe and effective. However, debate over the safety of silicone continues in the medical community. Many doctors avoid silicone because of its history of causing problems in some patients, including migration or shifting of the silicone, infection, and hardening.

Are You a Candidate for Fillers?

Because there are so many ways to fill different types of wrinkles and reshape facial contours, you and your physician will want to review the options together and select the treatments that will work best for you. It is a very customized process, and often a combination of different types of fillers will produce the best results.

If you have a history of allergy to meat or other bovine products, or severe allergies in general, you may not be a good candidate for bovine collagen. About three in one hundred people test positive for bovine allergy.

Your Filler Procedure

For virtually all the injectable fillers, no advance preparation is needed. The exception is a simple skin test to rule out the possibility of an allergic reaction to bovine collagen. After a tiny amount of the solution is injected in a location

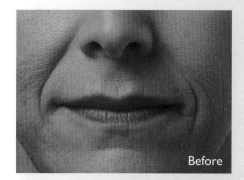
Before

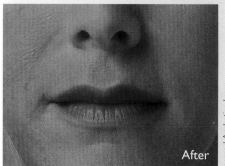
After

Inamed Aeshetics, Inc.

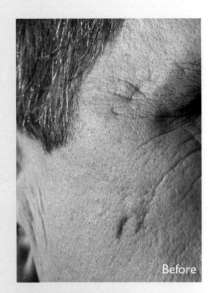
Before

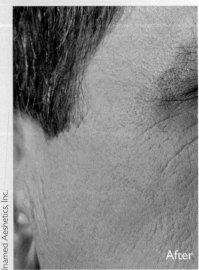
After

Collagen fills in scars and wrinkles.

elsewhere on your body, such as the arm, you'll need to watch the area closely for four to six weeks for signs of an allergic response, such as severe itching, swelling, or redness. Most reactions occur within three days, but the four-to-six-week window is necessary because a reaction could occur anytime during this period. To be certain, most doctors recommend a second allergy test two weeks after the first one.

Of course, if your doctor is using the newer hyaluronic acid, Restylane, allergic reaction will not be an issue. More and more doctors are using this acid as a soft tissue filler to reduce wrinkles.

Filler Injections

Once you and your doctor have decided where you would like to have fillers injected, the areas are cleaned with alcohol. Most fillers require an anesthetic, often a *nerve block anesthetic*. A nerve block is a deeper, more targeted injection of anesthetic into tissue containing sensory nerves in areas around the lips.

If you have concerns about pain, ask your doctor about anesthetics. If your chosen filler liquid is suitable for smaller needles, it may be possible to receive microinjections, which are less painful.

Filler Implants

Most implants used for wrinkles are produced in strips or threads, so each piece of material has two ends and is threaded through the area of tissue being filled. After the location for each incision is disinfected, a local anesthetic will be injected. Once the skin is numb, the doctor will make a tiny incision at each end of the crease or wrinkle. Then, with a special threading device, the implant material is pulled from one incision through to the other incision. Next, the ends are trimmed and a single, hair-thin stitch is placed at each end to hold the implant in place while the incisions heal. In some cases, a kind of suture is used that will simply fall out on its own. Otherwise, your doctor will need to remove the stitches in a few days.

The incisions' locations will vary, of course, with the location of the wrinkle or groove being filled. Basically, however, incisions are hidden at the top and bottom of the line or fold being treated.

After Your Procedure

Filler Injections

One of the reasons injection fillers are so popular is that the results are virtually instantaneous. The wrinkle or sunken area will be softened and less pronounced, and your face will be subtly redefined. For a few days, you may have a little temporary swelling or puffiness, so the result you first see in the mirror will improve once the swelling resolves. Some short-term redness is possible, too.

Your doctor will give you detailed instructions on how to care for your skin after your treatment. Because filler options vary so widely, the follow-up care varies, too. For most injections, you'll simply need to keep your face clean of cosmetics for a day. Ask your doctor if it's okay to apply a cold pack to reduce swelling. It's important to ask since you should not apply cold or heat to an area that has been treated with hyaluronic acids.

Filler Implants

A synthetic implant can reshape your face more distinctly than an injection. Swelling will usually be more pronounced with implants than with injections, but will be gone in a few days (and is rarely severe enough to make you want to hide at home for more than a day). Temporary bruising often appears on the skin above where an implant is placed, but this can be covered by makeup.

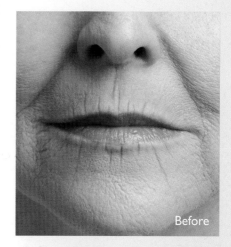

Before

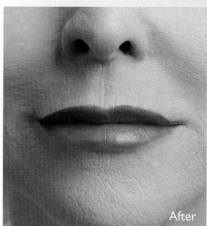

After

Inamed Aesthetics, Inc.

Collagen adds volume to the lips and adds definition to the border.

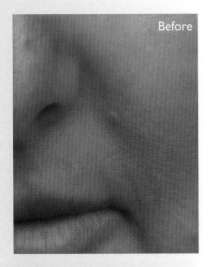
Before

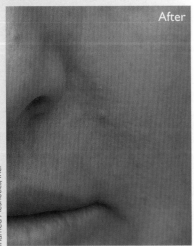
After

Hyaluronic acid is used to soften "marionette" lines, which run from the corners of the lips down toward the chin.

Inamed Aeshetics, Inc.

The improvement is seen immediately; however, the final, filled-in effect of your implants is normally apparent after about three months, when your own tissue growth has had time to make its contribution, too. You will notice that the treated areas of your face look firmer, with more defined contours. Where once there was a depression or deep groove, a smoother, younger-looking surface has appeared.

How Long Will Results Last?

As mentioned throughout this chapter, the results of temporary injectable wrinkle fillers can last anywhere from three months to a year. Some of the newer soft tissue fillers may last up to two years. These results vary from person to person, depending on how your own body responds to the substance. Overall, however, the definition of what's temporary for you largely depends on the depth of the area treated, how much material is injected, and how much of your own collagen and tissue repair your body produces. Again, this is variable, so your best guide will be what you observe in the mirror.

Permanent implant fillers are just that. Most of them will last longer than you do, unless for some reason you decide to have them removed. Occasionally, individuals request removal because they are not happy with how an implant looks, or are unusually sensitive to its feel. More often, people who feel a new sensation with an implant quickly adapt and soon do not even notice it.

Potential Risks

An allergic response to either bovine or donor collagen (derived from tissue banks) is possible, although allergy testing should forestall this problem. Now and then, filler treatments may produce a lumpy appearance in the skin.

As mentioned earlier, as autologous fat is reabsorbed by the body, it can sometimes happen in an irregular way, creating an uneven surface. Also, there is a risk of infection at the site where fat is harvested and at the injection site.

There is a small risk of inflammation or infection at the ends of thread-like implants where they meet the suture areas, but prophylactic (preventative) antibiotics may be prescribed to prevent this. Sometimes, an implant may later appear to have moved or shifted. If you sense this, see your doctor, who can remove and reinsert it.

Combining Filler Procedures with Other Procedures

Soft tissue fillers can be used to complement virtually any other cosmetic facial procedure. They are most commonly used to fill in nasolabial folds when facelifts are performed. Fillers may also be used to fill lines in the forehead when a browlift is done.

Questions to Ask the Surgeon

- What are your medical credentials?
- What type of filler treatment is appropriate for me?
- Do I need an allergy skin test?
- What kind of pain medication is available to me?
- How quickly will I recover?
- Can you show me before-and-after photos of other patients?
- How should I care for my skin before and after the filler?
- Should I stop taking my usual medications or supplements?

CHAPTER 11

CHIN & CHEEK IMPLANTS

11

CHIN & CHEEK IMPLANTS

*I*f nature gave you less-than-ideal facial bone structure—perhaps your chin recedes or your cheeks seem too flat or hollow—your facial features may not appear balanced. Well-defined cheekbones and a strong chin not only convey beauty and strength, they can also draw attention away from facial flaws that might otherwise be noticeable.

Facial implants will give you a safe and long-lasting way to strengthen chin or cheeks without extensive surgery. In the United States each year, facial cosmetic surgeons safely and successfully perform an estimated 30,000 chin implantations and 10,000 cheek implant procedures.

What Are Facial Implants?

Facial implants, most commonly done for the cheeks or chin, are materials that are shaped and inserted below the skin and muscles. Cheek implants will plump up the cheeks. Chin implantation, sometimes referred to as *mentoplasty*, *genioplasty*, or *chinplasty*, makes the chin look stronger and more prominent. For surgery to place solid implants into your face, your doctor will use carefully shaped materials to build up flat areas, giving you a more attractive, proportional, and youthful face. Facial implants are considered permanent unless, for some reason, you choose to have them removed.

Facial Implant Materials

Facial implants can be made out of bone, fat, or other tissue from your body (autologous tissue) or from a donor source. Besides human or animal tissue, metals (such as titanium), ceramic materials, and various types of synthetics have been used. Some are injectable—liquids or semiliquids available as pastes, gels, or oils. Injectable implants aren't usually as long-lasting or as effective as solid implants.

Most facial cosmetic surgeons prefer to use synthetic rather than *autologous* or donated tissue for several reasons. Synthetic implants come in all sizes, shapes, and strengths. They can be tailor-made for elasticity and durability. There's no need to remove tissue from other places on your body; thus the procedure doesn't take as long and is easier on you. Most synthetics can be custom-trimmed for the very best fit. And the capsule that forms around synthetic implants makes them relatively easy to remove in the unlikely event they need to be replaced.

The most common synthetic facial implant materials are the *polymers* silicone and *expanded polytetrafluoroethylene* (ePTFE, often sold as Gore-Tex), Polymers—giant molecules made up of smaller molecules—are sometimes referred to as "plastics," but they can be made of organic materials, such as rubber or cellulose, as well.

Silicone, a combination of the elements silicon and oxygen, is sometimes called "synthetic rubber," although it's more durable than natural rubber. Implanted in solid form in facial implants, silicone is strong and causes no toxic or allergic reactions. Most doctors consider silicone, as manufactured today, to be safe and long-lasting. Solid silicone implants have been safely and effectively used in facial implants since the 1960s.

A carbon-based polymer with hundreds of uses, ePTFE is prized for its water resistance and "breathability." In fact, ePTFE might be part of your wardrobe—in your hiking shoes or raincoat, for example. Like silicone, ePTFE is safe and long-lasting.

Are You a Candidate for a Facial Implant?

A chin implant can make a dramatic difference in the overall harmony of your facial features. Since a weak chin makes the nose appear bigger, patients seeking rhinoplasty—a much more extensive procedure—may find that with a chin implant the nose looks more normal in size.

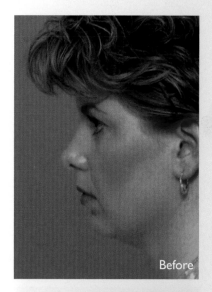
Before

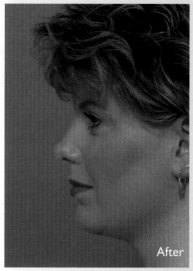
After

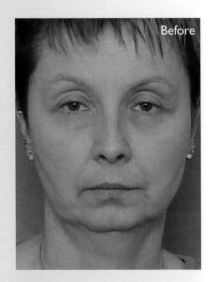
Before

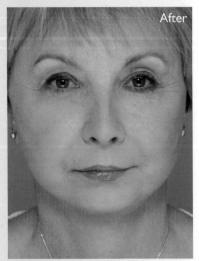
After

Chin implant with facelift. An implant improves the profile and also adds balance in a frontal view.

If your chin or cheeks are out of balance with the rest of your face and you're in good health, you may be an excellent candidate for facial implants. Age can be a factor; doctors generally prefer to perform facial implant surgery only on people who have reached adulthood, since bone growth (in teens, for example) can cause implants to shift.

Chin implantation is sometimes postponed and the patient referred to an oral surgeon or orthodontist if there is a severe underbite or overbite. If your incision will be in your mouth, be sure to tell your doctor about any dental or gum problems you might have. As with any surgery, you'll need to stop smoking well in advance of the procedure.

Your Facial Implant Procedure

Your doctor may have you prepare for surgery by using an antibacterial facial cleanser or mouthwash, depending on whether incisions will be external or intraoral, for a few days. You'll probably report to your doctor's office for surgery in the morning and go home soon after the operation. Cheek implants take 45 minutes to an hour; a chin implant as little as 20 minutes.

Your doctor will insert your cheek or chin implant using either an *intraoral approach,* inside the mouth, or an *external approach,* in which the incisions are made outside the mouth.

Intraoral Approach

Intraoral incisions for cheek implants will be made on the inside of your upper lip, between the cheek and the gums. For a chin implant, the intraoral incision will be near the bottom of the inside lower lip. The surgeon will create a pocket in the area of your face where the implant will go. The pocket will be just the right size to hold the implant and keep it from slipping. It is seldom necessary to attach the implant to underlying tissues or bone. Once the implant is in place, your body will grow tissue, creating a capsule that will hold the implant firmly in place. Nonetheless, some surgeons prefer to secure the implant with sterile permanent screws.

The intraoral approach leaves no visible scar, though some doctors believe it's harder to control infection than with the external approach. Either way, infection is unlikely if you follow your doctor's diet and hygiene instructions after surgery.

External Approach

With this approach, external incisions will be on the outside or inside of the lower eyelids for cheek implants. The approach allows for the most exact placement of the implants. If you're having cheek implants at the same time as eyelid surgery or a mid-face lift, for example, your doctor will probably use the same lower eyelid incisions.

For the chin, the external approach uses an incision just under your chin (*submental*), in an existing crease. Any scarring from external incisions, once healed, is generally noticeable only to you and your doctor.

As with the intraoral approach, your surgeon will create a pocket in facial tissue under the skin and muscle. During the procedure the surgeon will carefully measure the pocket in order to select the proper size and shape of the implant. The implant can be shaped, if necessary, before it is inserted.

Plastic surgeons take great care to ensure sterility and prevent infection, and never is this more important than when incisions are in the mouth. Your physician will take numerous protective measures, which may include the following:

- Giving you intravenous antibiotics throughout the procedure.

- Rinsing the pocket with an antibacterial solution.

- Not allowing the implant to come in contact with mouth fluids or skin.

- Changing surgical gloves before placing the implant.

- Not touching the implant at all, even with a gloved hand.

Once the implants are in place, the surgeon will close the incisions using dissolving sutures in the mouth or small, removable external sutures. If you had cheek implants,

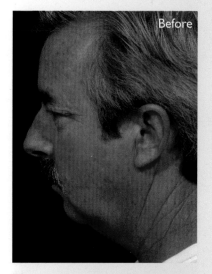
Before

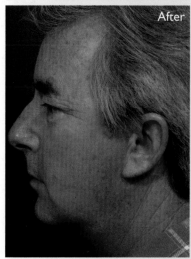
After

In addition to chin implant, this patient had a facelift.

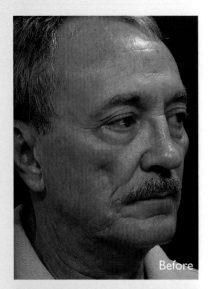

Before

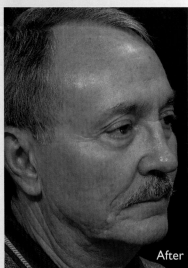

After

After cheek inplants.

your cheeks may be lightly bandaged. After chin augmentation, the chin is generally taped to minimize swelling and discomfort and to hold the implant in place.

After Your Facial Implant Procedure

After your cheek or chin implant, you'll have some postsurgical swelling, but you will see results instantly. Your face will have fuller, more balanced, natural contours—the "good bones" you may not have been born with. You'll have a stronger, more attractive profile, and you'll feel better about the way you look. Your doctor will probably use synthetic implants that retain their structure and shape, so it's unlikely you'll ever need to have them replaced.

If the incisions are in your mouth, your surgeon will give you specific instructions for diet and oral hygiene. He or she may recommend using an antiseptic mouthwash with warm water several times a day and not using a toothbrush near the incisions.

Side Effects, Risks, and Complications

Your face will feel stiff at first, so moving your mouth—smiling, talking, eating, and laughing, for example—might be difficult and a bit uncomfortable for several days. Your doctor will probably prescribe a soft diet for the first few days.

If your incisions are in your mouth, there will be no visible scars. External incisions will leave small, thin, white scars, but your doctor will have placed these incisions where the scars will not be noticeable.

The chance of complications with implant surgery is very low—under one percent. If your surgeon has successfully performed many such procedures, your risk is even lower. Your doctor, however, will explain the risks of your particular procedure. Very rare complications include shifting, *extrusion* (the implant projecting out of its pocket), or *malposition* (incorrect placement of the implant). To prevent these complications, your surgeon will customize the implant's size to fit snugly in the pocket. Heavy scarring can sometimes push an implant out of position, but this is extremely unlikely if you are not prone to keloid or hypertrophic scarring.

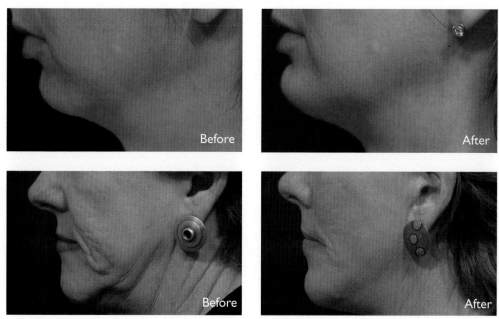

Bottom photos show chin implant combined with facelift and laser skin resurfacing around the mouth.

Questions to Ask the Surgeon

- How long will my implant last?
- Can my implant be removed if necessary?
- Where will my incisions be?
- If you insert the implant through my mouth, is there a greater risk of infection?
- Which implant material will you use? What are its advantages and disadvantages?

Combining Implant Surgery with Other Procedures

Cheek and chin implants may be done at the same time. Each of these procedures can also be performed with facelifts, rhinoplasty, eyelid surgery, browlifts, and skin resurfacing.

Though cheek implants can be done along with a facelift, they might instead *delay* the need for a facelift. Besides restoring fullness to your cheeks, these implants sometimes lift sagging tissues and smooth the lines between your nose and mouth. In patients with a great deal of sagging in the midface, however, cheek implants might not provide enough lift and smoothness and a facelift or midface lift may be more helpful.

CHAPTER 12

LIP AUGMENTATION

12

LIP AUGMENTATION

*A*s we get older, our lips may become wrinkled and lose volume as tissues shrink. Even if you were blessed with beautiful lips, you may find your lips are losing some of their fullness. Facial plastic surgeons can add volume and smoothness to lips that are too thin, too flat, or too wrinkled.

With today's options you can add lip volume that lasts longer than a few hours or days. Temporary and semipermanent injectable substances are available for augmenting your lips, as well as surgical implants, the most lasting solution.

What Is Lip Augmentation?

Cosmetic *lip augmentation* is a medical procedure to make your lips larger, fuller, and more attractive. The term usually refers to injecting or surgically implanting a substance to smooth, fill out, reshape, and enhance the lips. Some lip augmentation procedures will also help correct wrinkles around the lips. Your procedure may be temporary, semipermanent, or long-lasting.

Lip augmentation may involve the whole lip or only the *vermillion*—the visible part of the actual lip, which is of course darker than skin surrounding the mouth. The lip's edge, where it meets the facial skin, is called the *vermillion border*. The double curve of the upper lip is often referred to as the *Cupid's bow*.

The type of procedure you have and the materials used will depend on the desired results, your own facial anatomy, and your doctor's experience. You may want to have just one lip augmented, though it's more common to do both lips to ensure the proper proportions.

Lip Augmentation Materials

Injectable Fillers

Injectable fillers can give you quick and dramatic results. Bovine collagen (from cow skin) may be the most well-known temporary filler. Collagen from cows and pigs is similar to human collagen—a protein that supports your skin, soft tissues, and bones.

Such temporary fillers can last from a few weeks to several months. If you opt for collagen injections, for example, you'll have to repeat them every couple of months to retain your full-lipped look. That may be a good way to go if you want to experiment with different looks before committing to a more permanent procedure.

Surgical Implants

Synthetic Implants

Synthetic lip implants are the most durable form of lip augmentation. They will plump up your lips without exaggerating their size. It may take you a while to get used to the feeling of solid implants in your lips, though the newest implant products are softer and more flexible than the older types.

Your surgeon will probably use a form of expanded polytetrafluoroethylene (ePTFE), a synthetic substance derived from carbon. Gore-Tex™ and Teflon™ are well-known ePTFE materials. Newer implants, such as Advanta™, are improvements on Gore-Tex implants. Advanta, the leader in soft-tissue implants for the face, is the softest ePTFE implant available and does the best job of integrating with existing facial tissues.

Biological Implants

Biological implants can be fashioned from many of the body's tissues, including skin, fat, fascia, and tendons. The look and feel can be quite natural. Called autologous, meaning the tissue comes from one's own body, these implants are long-lasting;

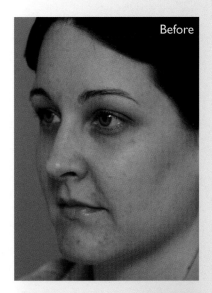
Before

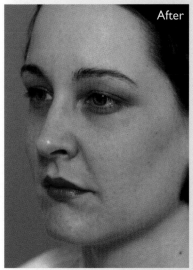
After

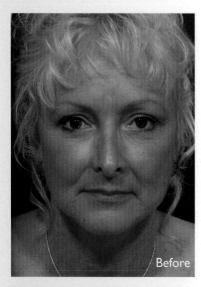

Before

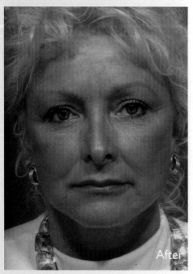

After

however, most of the substance will eventually be absorbed by your body. As a result, the procedure will have to be repeated at regular intervals.

Autologous implants, often processed from fat removed from the abdomen by liposuction, are more complex than most other types of lip augmentation implant surgery. The reason is that two procedures are needed, one to remove the fat and the other to implant it. Still, an advantage of human-tissue implants is that there's almost no risk your body will reject them.

Similarly, donor tissues are processed and purified, so the risk of infection or disease transmission also is low. Alloderm™ is the brand name for donor skin that's specially processed and then precut in various sizes for implantation. Alloderm implants are soft and feel natural, and since your own cells will grow into the implants, the effect is long-lasting—often two years or more.

Other Lip Procedures

Laser lip rejuvenation does not enlarge the lips, but it can smooth out lines and wrinkles on and around them. Botox injections are sometimes used to augment the effect of fillers; chemical peels may achieve similar results.

A *lip lift* is surgery to remove a strip of skin beneath the nose, shortening the distance between the nasal columella and the upper lip. This procedure also makes the vermillion more visible. The incision is hidden at the base of the nose and is closed with tiny absorbable sutures, which disappear in about a week.

Other procedures bring tissue from the inside to the outside of the lips. *Lip advancement*, for example, elevates and reshapes the inner lip lining to enlarge the vermillion.

Lip lifts and advancement are more complicated than implant procedures and the recovery time is longer. Your doctor will recommend the best technique for you based on your unique features, your goals, and your medical history.

Are You a Candidate?

If you're a healthy man or woman of almost any age and you'd like to have fuller, smoother lips, you could be a candidate for lip augmentation. These days, the number of lip augmentation patients ages 19 to 34 is about the same as in those ages 35 to 50.

Before lip augmentation surgery, your teeth and gums should be in good condition. Necessary dental work should be done well in advance of your surgery. Ask your plastic surgeon how long you should wait after dental work to have lip augmentation surgery. Some experts believe that even minor dental work such as a cleaning releases bacteria and can make you more vulnerable to infection after your surgery.

People who have recurrent oral herpes (cold sores) should postpone surgery if the herpes is active. Some doctors will not perform lip augmentation on anyone with a history of recurrent oral herpes because the surgery may activate the virus. Tell your doctor if you have severe allergies, including an allergy to lidocaine, a local anesthetic that's part of some augmentation products. If a skin test is required for the implant you want and you're found to be allergic to the substance, your doctor will help you choose another implant material.

Your Lip Augmentation Procedure

Filler Lip Injections

Injections for lip augmentation are usually done in the doctor's office. Many patients report little or no pain, so there is often no need for anesthesia. Furthermore, the injectable materials also contain Lidocaine, which helps numb the tissues. If anesthesia is required, a local anesthetic is used. It can take a series of twelve to sixteen injections of the filler to complete the job.

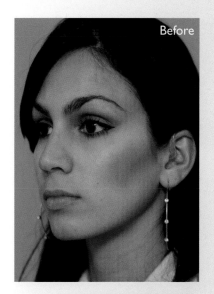

Before

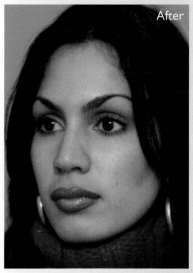

After

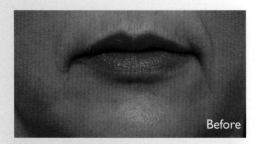

Before

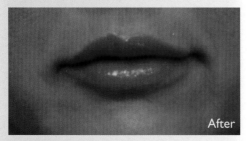

After

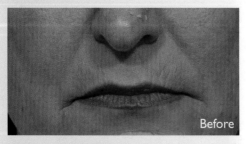

Before

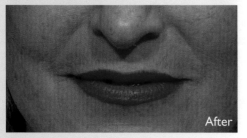

After

Lip Implants

The procedure will most likely be performed under local anesthesia in your doctor's office or surgical suite. The procedure usually takes 30 to 90 minutes. Since the mouth tends to harbor bacteria, great care will be taken to ensure sterility.

For the typical implantation procedure, your doctor will numb your lips, then make four small incisions at the corners of the upper and lower lips. Through these incisions small tunnels will be formed. The implant material will be rolled or shaped to the proper size, pulled through the tunnels, and trimmed for the best fit. The incisions will then be sutured shut, usually with dissolving stitches.

You'll probably start taking antibiotics a few days before your lip implant surgery. This will protect against infection in the area where the implant will be inserted.

After Your Lip Augmentation Procedure

You'll see results immediately, though your lips will be swollen at first. With most injectables, you can go back to work the next day.

If you have had surgically placed implants, you'll require a recovery period of a week or more. That's because, no matter how careful you are, it's impossible not to move your lips. It's important to get enough rest, give yourself sufficient time off from work and other activities, and follow your doctor's instructions, which will probably include diet recommendations and directions for oral and facial hygiene. If you didn't see your dentist before your lip augmentation procedure, ask your doctor how long you should wait after surgery before having dental work.

Drink plenty of water and apply ointment approved by your doctor to your lips. Use sterile cotton swabs. Avoid applying any creams, ointments, lotions, and other substances to the incisions unless instructed by your doctor. Don't touch your mouth or incisions with your hands or allow anyone else to do so.

As much as possible, avoid talking, laughing, chewing, even smiling. Soft foods will give your mouth a needed rest—but don't drink through a straw and don't eat or drink anything hot. When you start eating solid foods again, thoroughly wash fresh fruits and vegetables and make sure meat and fish are well cooked.

Wear lipstick or other products that contain sunscreen. Why? The skin on your lips has fewer layers than your body's skin and is less effective at retaining moisture. Also, the lips produce less melanin, skin pigment, than the skin on the rest of your body. *Melanin* is the body's natural reaction to the sun—it darkens the skin to screen out ultraviolet rays. Since your lips don't have the same protection, experts recommend that you always wear a clear or tinted lip product with an SPF of at least 15.

Side Effects, Risks, and Complications

At first, there may be slight bruising around the mouth, or your lips might look darker or paler than usual. Because surgery will disturb some facial muscles and nerves, normal, everyday things like smiling and talking might feel strange for a while. You may have trouble drinking and eating, even with the soft-food diet your doctor will recommend.

Depending on the type and size of implant, you may be able to feel it from the outside. This side effect, called *palpability*, was more common with older, firmer implants. The newer products, as noted earlier, are softer and feel more natural. Your lips may be quite dry at first and some of the skin may peel.

There's a very slight risk that the implants will move out of position (*migrate*) and that the lips will look asymmetrical or lumpy. There's also a small possibility of *extrusion*, when the implant works its way out of the pocket and sometimes protrudes through the skin. Call your doctor's office right away if the implant seems to be shifting.

Questions to Ask Your Doctor

- How can I be sure my lips won't be too full after augmentation?

- Will I be sedated during the procedure? Should I plan for someone to drive me home?

- Do you recommend massaging the incision sites to promote healing? If so, what's the best and safest technique?

- Can my implants be easily replaced if necessary?

- How long will my lip augmentation results last?

- How far in advance of lip augmentation surgery should I schedule dental work? How soon after lip augmentation surgery may I schedule dental work?

CHAPTER 13

SKIN REJUVENATION

13

SKIN REJUVENATION

*M*ore youthful skin is less than a millimeter away.

Under the top layers of facial skin—which may bear signs of sun damage, aging, acne, or superficial scarring—lies a younger-looking skin. Cosmetic skin resurfacing removes the upper layers to reveal the soft, smooth, fresh, healthier-looking skin underneath. The most effective and lasting skin-resurfacing techniques are laser skin resurfacing and chemical peels.

What Is Laser Skin Resurfacing?

Laser skin resurfacing is just that—a resurfacing of the facial skin, erasing fine lines and wrinkles. Lasers can also eliminate imperfections such as age spots, spider veins, excess facial hair, and cherry angiomas, which resemble blood-filled pimples. How does a laser work on the skin? A laser produces a narrow beam of light that emits an intense heat. Targeted at the skin, the laser can eliminate or reduce skin imperfections in a fraction of a second without damaging surrounding tissue. Because the laser beam is computer-driven, the depth of the beam's penetration into the skin is controlled.

Two basic types of lasers are used to treat skin: *ablative* and *nonablative*. Ablative lasers, the more aggressive of the two, are capable of ablating, or completely removing, a layer of skin. Nonablative lasers are less aggressive and are used for removing skin flaws such as age spots or excess facial hair.

Skin Resurfacing with Ablative Lasers

Using ablative lasers is the most dramatic way of restoring the skin's youthful appearance. Laser resurfacing removes moderate to severe sun damage, leaving remarkably smoother, brighter, and firmer skin. The laser heat also tightens underlying tissues, creating firmer skin. As a result, ablative lasers soften the edges of wrinkles and dramatically diminish deep crow's feet or upper lip lines. When lasers are used to resurface the skin, they also can soften the appearance of minor facial scars by as much as 50 to 60 percent.

Are You a Candidate for Ablative Laser Treatment?

Ablative laser skin resurfacing is a more serious procedure than nonablative resurfacing, so your doctor will carefully evaluate your general health and ability to tolerate the removal of a layer of skin. You are not a candidate if you have a current skin infection, have a previous history of severe scarring, or have used Accutane within the last year or two. Unstable diabetes or autoimmune disorders also rule out laser resurfacing for most people.

To maximize the benefits of any laser treatment, stay out of the sun and be extra vigilant about applying a daily high-SPF sunscreen for two weeks before your procedure, as well as forever after!

Your Ablative Laser Procedure

Before laser resurfacing, be sure to discuss your medical history fully with your doctor. It's particularly important to let your doctor know if you have a history of cold sores, herpes, or other viral skin infections, as you will need to take antiviral medications both before your procedure and during the healing period to prevent a new outbreak.

Ablative laser skin resurfacing is not an invasive surgery in the same way a facelift is; however, it is an aggressive form of skin rejuvenation. Therefore, the procedure

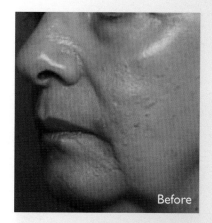

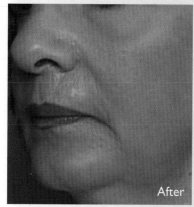

Laser skin resurfacing.

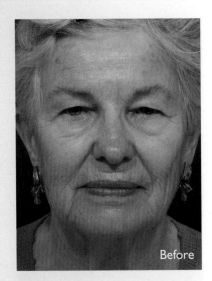

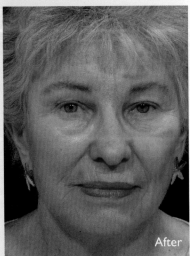

Laser resurfacing, along with eyelid lift and facelift.

must be performed in an operating room or surgical suite. You will be hooked up to a heart monitor, and a blood pressure cuff. Because the anesthetics used can stimulate the heart, routine monitoring is required. You'll also wear a small device, a pulse oximeter, on your index finger to monitor your blood oxygen level.

To guard against infection, your skin will be cleansed with disinfectant, and you'll be covered with sterile drapes. You'll also be wearing special goggles or eye shields to protect your eyes from the laser light.

Depending on the procedure, your doctor may apply a topical anesthetic. More often, ablative resurfacing requires either an injected nerve block or twilight sedation, which is given through an IV. When extensive work is needed, general anesthesia is sometimes recommended.

As the treatment starts, the doctor will use an instrument about the size of a pencil to pass the laser beam over your skin, removing the epidermis and part of the upper dermis. Because the laser is fully computerized, your doctor can precisely control the amount of energy in the beam, the density of the light, and the length of time it stays on your skin. Depending on your skin's condition and the areas to be treated, the procedure will take from 30 minutes to over an hour. Some parts of the face may require a second pass; your doctor will carefully avoid letting the laser's light penetrate too deeply. In many cases, as doctors treat the skin surface, they also see the skin firming up as the laser is passed across the face.

When the ablative resurfacing is complete, your face will be wrapped either in an antibiotic-soaked gauze bandage or in a mask-like dressing that resembles plastic wrap. Many surgeons use autologous platelet gel on the lasered skin to help accelerate healing.

You'll rest in a recovery area for a few hours until any lingering light-headedness from the sedation or anesthesia has worn off. Then you'll need a friend or relative to drive you home.

After Your Ablative Laser Procedure

In the first few days your face will be quite red and will be swollen. You'll be wearing the dressings on your face for several days. It is important that you wear these because they help your skin retain moisture and prevent exposure to the air, which might encourage scabs to form and cause scarring. You may be asked to return to the doctor's office several times for dressing changes; however, some of the newest coverings can remain up to one week, avoiding the need to change the dressing.

Full recovery from ablative resurfacing is lengthy and can take two to six weeks. Still, most women can apply makeup in about two weeks; most can return to work around this time. Men usually grow their beards for two to three weeks, which helps camouflage their pink skin. For both sexes the pinkness gradually fades over the next two to three months. How quickly it does so is dependent on the regimen the physician recommends to the patient (skin care products both pre- and post-treatment) and how closely the patient follows it. Recovery times vary widely.

After the dressings and ointments are gone, you'll see much softer, pinker, and smoother skin. Most lines and wrinkles will be radically reduced if not eliminated entirely, along with roughness and pigmentation spots. During the next several months, the changes generated by new collagen formation will slowly appear. Your skin will appear firmer and tighter, in many cases dramatically so.

You'll be visiting your doctor again a few days to a week after your procedure to have the dressings removed, and you'll be given specific instructions for your follow-up care. Pain is generally minimal, and most patients use narcotics for only one day, if at all. To further the healing process, you will want to take the following steps:

■ Sleep on two pillows for a week or two to reduce swelling.

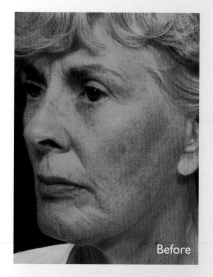
Before

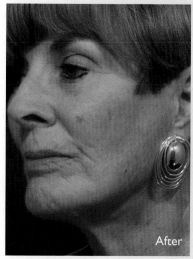
After

Four months after skin resurfacing with ablative laser.

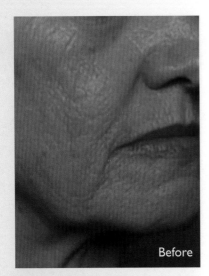

Before

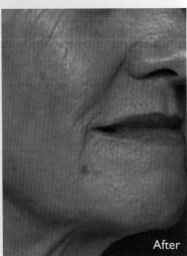

After

Several months after ablative laser skin resurfacing.

- Follow the detailed instructions from your doctor on how to apply the ointments and replace the protective dressings. Do not remove the dressings unless you have been instructed to do so.

- Wash your face several times a day with a gentle warm-water spray and the soap your doctor provides (unless you have an extended dressing in place).

- Take any other medications, antibiotics or antiviral medications your doctor has prescribed for you.

- Become a sunscreen zealot—safeguard your new skin with generous daily applications of a high-quality, high-SPF sunscreen.

Depending on the depth of your treatment, your healing time may vary from one to several weeks. If you have a medium depth laser resurfacing, you may be able to return to work wearing makeup after only one week.

How Long Will Results Last?

With proper skin care and sun protection, the results of a complete resurfacing in most cases will last a minimum of five years, and for many people even eight or ten years. As the aging process continues, you will see gradual changes appear. It is not unusual to repeat a complete ablative resurfacing, but your doctor can offer a variety of complementary treatments to prolong the renewed appearance of your skin.

Potential Risks

Ablative laser resurfacing, because it exposes a raw new layer, introduces the same risk of infection as any technique that removes a significant depth of skin. Proper follow-up care can protect you from the possibility of infection. If there is undiagnosed herpes simplex virus (HSV) present in the skin, it may be activated by the laser and produce scarring.

Lasers Used in Skin Rejuvenation	
Ablative Lasers	
Carbon dioxide (CO2)	Renews severely sun-weathered skin by resurfacing the upper layer. Softens the edges of wrinkles and dramatically diminishes deep crow's feet or upper lip lines.
"Superpulsed" CO2	Renews severely sun-weathered skin by resurfacing the upper layer. Softens the edges of wrinkles, dramatically diminishes deep crow's feet or upper lip lines.
Erbium:YAG	Resurfaces the top layer of skin and tightens underlying tissue. Stimulates the growth of collagen, further diminishing fine lines and wrinkles from mild to moderate sun damage. Improves minor surface scars and splotchy discoloration.
Nonablative Lasers	
Neodymium	Also known as Nd:YAG. Laser improves skin firmness and elasticity. Popular version, Cool Touch™, uses unique cooling spray that soothes sensitive nerve endings while the laser does its work. Nd:YAG laser is also effective for removing unwanted dark pigment and unwanted hair.
Yellow Light (Pulsed-Dye)	Effectively removes port-wine stains, rosacea, and enlarged blood vessels. Also treats some raised scars and removes red, orange, and yellow tattoo pigments.
Alexandrite and Ruby	Alexandrite laser is effective for hair removal in people with darker skin. Ruby laser works best on those with pale skin and dark hair. Both are used in tattoo removal. Alexandrite targets black, blue, and green; Ruby removes black, purple, violet, and other dark colors.
Diode	Removes hair in people with fair skin and dark hair. Also known as Diolite™, this laser is effective in treating facial spider veins and flat brown spots.
Intense Pulsed Light	Not a true laser, but effective in long-term hair removal, treatment of brown spots, and superficial broken blood vessels. Rather than single wavelengths, intense pulsed light uses all the visible wavelengths. Controls allow physician to change a colored filter in the device, so light can be adapted for individual problems and skin types. Treatment also useful for premature mild wrinkling.

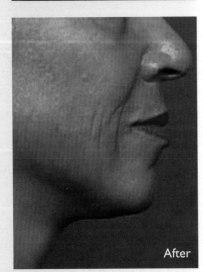

Before

After

Five months after ablative laser skin resurfacing.

Are You a Candidate for Laser Treatment?

Laser treatments work best on people with fair skin that is relatively oily, although other skin types have been successfully treated. Only your doctor can determine whether your skin is appropriate for a specific type of laser procedure.

Treating the Skin with Nonablative Lasers

These lasers treat skin imperfections by destroying defects caused by tissues beneath the skin, leaving surface layers undamaged. Accordingly, there is no wound to the skin surface and healing time is minimal. These lasers are used to make a variety of cosmetic improvements.

Nonablative laser resurfacing also causes the collagen layer just beneath the epidermis to gradually thicken, which firms and tones the skin. This helps eliminate finer lines and wrinkles such as those around the eyes, upper lip, cheeks, and forehead. Although you'll need a series of treatments, depending on your skin's condition, downtime is minimal compared to ablative resurfacing. For this reason, many patients prefer these more frequent, but less aggressive treatments. However, if your skin is heavily damaged, an ablative procedure may be the best option.

Other uses for the nonablative laser include the removal of age spots, dark skin splotches, spider veins, port-wine birthmarks, warts, and excess facial hair. Laser hair removal is most effective on dark hair. Why? The laser targets only dark melanin pigment within or near a hair follicle. Blonde, red, and gray hair follicles lack this pigment, so laser hair removal isn't effective for them. A nonablative laser treatment may also offer some improvement, perhaps 10 to 20 percent, to facial scars.

If you have laser hair removal scheduled, you'll need to stop plucking or waxing for four to six weeks in advance. And don't shave for several days before your appointment, as the stubble will help your doctor guide the laser's direction.

Your Nonablative Laser Procedure

These procedures can be done in the doctor's office. Most nonablative laser procedures are performed by a member of the doctor's staff, often a technician. You'll lie on a table or recline in a dental-style chair, usually with a simple gown or medical smock over your clothing. You'll wear protective eye goggles or eye shields.

Your need for any anesthetic will vary depending on the complexity of your skin problem and your pain tolerance. A fairly superficial age spot, for example, will normally produce brief strong stinging but nothing intense enough to require a numbing cream. If you are having a blood vessel or deep pigment area corrected, you may require either an injection of lidocaine or a topical cream, which should numb the area in about 20 minutes. Ask your doctor what kind of pain relief would be most appropriate for you.

After your skin is cleansed, your doctor will pass the laser's handpiece over the affected area on your face. You may occasionally hear a sharp "pop." This noise is simply the sound of the laser fizzling a hair within a follicle. These follicles are present in many parts of your skin, even where you have only light, barely visible facial hairs.

These procedures usually take from 15 to 45 minutes, depending on how much of your face is being treated. Afterward, you may be given a cold gel pack to place over your face for a few minutes to cool any residual burning you may feel.

After Your Nonablative Laser Procedure

If you've had a blood vessel or a pigmented area such as an age spot or tattoo removed, the skin will immediately turn white and then change to a reddish-purple color about five to ten minutes after the treatment. Mild swelling is possible, but normally not enough to be noticeable to anyone else. Your skin color will gradually return to normal over a one- to two-week period. You can disguise it with makeup in the meantime. With intense pulsed light treatments for rosacea, spider veins, or age spots, there is usually no change in skin color after a treatment.

What Do Nonablative Lasers Do?

- Firm and tone the skin
- Remove age spots or melasma
- Remove spider veins
- Remove port-wine birthmarks
- Reduce rosacea reddening
- Remove unwanted hair
- Lessen acne scars, other minor scars
- Remove warts
- Remove tattoos

In most cases, nonablative laser sessions require minimal follow-up. The basics include not picking or scratching at the skin while any discoloration remains, and faithfully using a high-SPF sunblock. If you choose to wear makeup afterward, ask your doctor what kind is appropriate, and apply and remove it very gently.

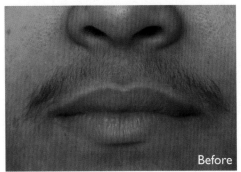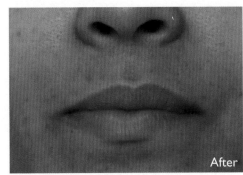

Several laser treatments are often required to permanently remove excess facial hair.

Although it often takes a series of six to ten nonablative treatments to achieve the best results, once a vascular or pigment problem is corrected, the result is permanent. However, if your aim was simply to counteract overall mild sun damage, you may decide on an additional series of treatments after several years to treat continuing sun damage and aging. For ongoing permanent hair removal, you may need touch-up sessions a few years later, as new hair follicles continue to develop.

Potential Risks

Nonablative laser treatments are considered extremely safe. However, as with any procedure, scarring can occur in some individuals. If you are in the care of an experienced physician, the risk is very small. Proper screening to be sure you do not have a history of severe scarring is important. Rarely, white spots or other pigmentation problems can appear after laser treatments, particularly in people with dark or olive-toned skin.

What Is a Chemical Peel?

A chemical peel is a procedure in which a chemical solution is applied to remove the top layer of the facial skin, leaving your face smoother and fresher. Peels restore sun-damaged skin. They also diminish wrinkles, acne scars, and can improve irregularities in the skin tone. For example, a peel can eliminate discoloration such as *melasma*, the brown patches that often accompany pregnancy. Peels will also eliminate age spots and the yellowish bumps called *solar elastosis*, which are areas of degenerated collagen caused by sun exposure. Peels can remove the often precancerous lesions known as *actinic keratoses*.

Although a chemical peel can soften the appearance of deep wrinkles, such as nasolabial folds and frown lines, it will not remove them. A peel won't tighten skin, but because it improves its surface and texture, your skin may appear firmer. Some research indicates that peels boost collagen production, which may help forestall the formation of new wrinkles.

Modern formulas for chemical peels contain a blend of ingredients that offer additional benefits. For example, a peel formula may contain hormones, anti-acne agents, or melanin inhibitors. Hormones enhance the plumpness of the skin by increasing moisture content. Anti-acne ingredients kill bacteria and absorb excess oils. Melanin inhibitors help prohibit the formation of skin discoloration or brown spots.

Types of Peels

Light Peels

The most popular peel is the *light peel* or *superficial peel*. These peels remove the top layer of skin—the dead surface cells called the *stratum corneum*. The chemical solutions in these peels are *alpha hydroxy acids* (AHA), most of which are derived from citrus fruits, milk sugars, and sugar cane. The mildest of the peel formulas, AHAs brighten, freshen, and exfoliate skin, repairing minor sun damage and smoothing dry

Chemical Peels Improve:

- Fine lines and wrinkles
- Uneven pigmentation
- Shallow acne scars
- Sun-damaged skin
- Age spots
- Freckling

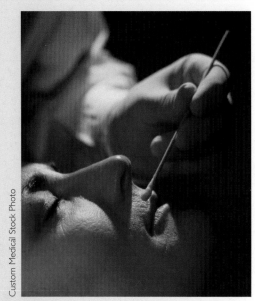

Application of chemical peel solution.

areas. Because AHAs remove only the most superficial layer of the skin, healing is so swift that these are sometimes called "weekend" peels. Many people will have a light peel done on a Friday and return to work on Monday, with minimal makeup. Many people will have a series of these peels.

Medium Peels

For a *medium peel,* a more potent chemical is used to remove all of the outer skin layer, or epidermis. The chemical, *trichloroacetic acid* (TCA) is a colorless synthetic acid, normally used in a concentration of about 35 percent. Because it penetrates more deeply than a light peel, a medium peel goes further to rejuvenate sun-damaged skin. Medium peels also reduce fine surface lines and wrinkles, often completely removing them. A medium peel is particularly effective at treating uneven pigment, such as age spots or melasma. It will also diminish superficial blemishes and shallow scarring from acne, but not deep pitted scars.

Depending on your skin's condition and what you'd like to have treated, your doctor may combine your medium peel with a simultaneous light peel. After the AHA exfoliates the most superficial layer of your skin, the TCA penetrates more deeply, maximizing the benefits.

Deep Peels or Modified Deep Peels

The traditional deep peel procedure, which you may have heard about, uses a chemical called *phenol* or carbolic acid. A *deep peel* removes all of the epidermis and part of the skin's middle layer, the dermis. As a result, it removes wrinkles around the mouth and eyes. Creases in the nasolabial fold and deep crow's feet soften but do not disappear totally.

Because phenol is such a powerful chemical, it makes the traditional deep peel a serious medical procedure. Why? The chemical solution can be difficult to control, and if it penetrates too deeply it can cause scarring and pigmentation problems.

Furthermore, if the phenol solution penetrates into the blood stream, it can cause heart rhythm disturbances or kidney damage.

Since the risks, recovery, and complications are much higher with a traditional phenol peel, it is rarely done anymore. A newer procedure, a *modified deep peel*, is rapidly growing in popularity. For this procedure the peel solution ingredients—liquid soap, Croton oil, phenol, and water—are modified. The modification uses more Croton oil and only a small amount of phenol, which enhances the effect while eliminating the complications and potential toxicity frequently associated with the phenol peels.

You may hear this newer peel referred to as a Hetter Peel, named for Dr. Gregory Hetter, its inventor; a Croton oil peel; or a modified phenol peel. The effects of a modified deep peel are dramatic when used for facial wrinkling, especially the leathery crisscross lines, and the deep lines around the lips so common with sun damage. These peels also improve acne scarring and eliminate pigmentation problems.

The modified peel can be done on the entire face for an overall skin rejuvenation, or only in localized areas such as under the eyes for "crepey" lower lids or around the mouth to remove the vertical smoker's lines.

Are You a Candidate for a Peel?

If you simply want to smooth and refresh tired-looking skin, you're likely a candidate for a light peel performed at a qualified surgeon's office. Likewise, if you have dark or black skin, your best choice is a light peel, because it is less likely to cause any pigmentation change. Most people can work these peels into their schedules with minimal time off from work.

If you're fair-skinned, you may also be a good candidate for a medium peel. For medium-toned or dark skin there is some risk of irregular pigmentation, however. Be

> *Choose an aesthetic surgeon who specializes in the procedure you desire. A well-trained and highly competent surgeon should be kind, warm, and professional. The surgeon and his or her staff should be easy to talk to. Your entire experience should be a positive one.*
>
> — Dr. Kriston Kent

aware that healing can take up to two weeks, so you may want to plan a short vacation around your scheduled procedure.

Modified deep peels are recommended only for people with fair skin—they are not advisable for medium, dark, black, or very oily skin. Recovery may take one to two weeks, with redness lasting up to six months.

Preparing for Your Peel

If you are using Retin-A™ (retinoic acid) or a similar product as part of a skin care regimen, you should stop using it for two to three days prior to your peel. The technician doing the peel should be made aware of your Retin-A use since it will affect the penetration of the peel solution. Otherwise, cleansing is the only preparation needed for a light peel. You simply wash your face with the cleanser provided at your doctor's office when you arrive.

For a medium peel or modified deep peel, your doctor may recommend that you pretreat your skin for several weeks with a prescription cream such as Retin-A. This exfoliates the skin and allows the solution to penetrate more deeply. Your doctor will instruct you on whether you need to discontinue using the Retin-A before your peel. If one of your problems is dark spots or blotchiness, a bleaching cream, *hydroquinone*, might also be added to boost your skin's pretreatment conditioning. This cream suppresses the melanin in the skin, causing dark spots to lighten. Using the cream also lessens the risk of pigmentation problems after the peel. If you tend to get cold sores, your doctor will prescribe prophylactic (preventative) antiviral medications to suppress any new outbreak, which might spread from the lips into a treated facial area.

Before a modified deep peel, you'll need a medical checkup. Any deep peel patient who plans to undergo intravenous sedation should be checked for heart or renal (kidney) problems since the procedure carries a slightly increased risk for those with heart or kidney problems.

Stop smoking for at least a week before your appointment, and avoid alcohol. Both will impede healing—smoking constricts blood vessels and alcohol dehydrates your tissues, which need their natural fluids for repair. Start taking your antibiotics as instructed. These are prescribed because a modified deep peel leaves dermal tissue exposed, and as with any wound to the skin, it's important to prevent infection. Arrange for someone to drive you home afterward and help you for 24 to 48 hours; you may be light headed from the residual anesthesia.

Before a medium or modified deep peel, your doctor may have you stop certain medications for several weeks. *Anticoagulant*, or blood thinning, medicines or herbal supplements may make it harder to recover because your blood brings healing nutrients to the raw skin. Most doctors also recommend that if you're taking drugs known as *oral retinoids,* used to treat skin conditions such as severe acne or psoriasis, you stop these for six months before a deep peel. These drugs, which include Accutane, can slow new skin formation and increase the risk of scarring.

Your Peel Procedure

All peels involve solutions applied to the skin, but details vary according to the type of peel. Every peel is applied with attention to your individual skin tone, condition, and level of damage. Your doctor will carefully control the depth of penetration for the best results.

Usually, peels are done on the entire face. With the deeper peels, the depth of the peel is usually greater around the eyes and mouth since more wrinkles are usually present in these areas. Sometimes partial peels, or subunits of the face, are done when only a portion of the facial skin is damaged and in need of repair. However, such a partial peel may leave a line of demarcation between the treated and untreated regions.

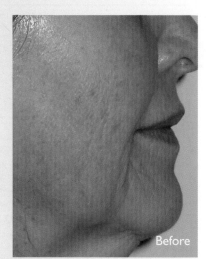
Before

Note mottled skin and fine wrinkles.

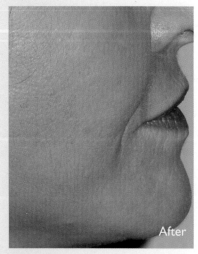
After

After modified deep peel combined with facelift

Light Peel

A light peel is performed in your doctor's office. After you've washed your face, your doctor or a well-trained medical staff member uses a solvent such as alcohol or diluted acetone to remove every remaining trace of makeup or oil. In some practices the doctor may pretreat your skin with a simple, painless procedure called *dermaplaning,* which lightly abrades the skin surface to remove dead skin cells and aid in the penetration of the chemicals. This is usually done by passing a bladed instrument that resembles an electric razor over your skin. Some doctors use a blade, similar to a scalpel.

Then the AHA solution is evenly applied, usually with a cotton pad or brush. You'll feel stinging, but it is usually not uncomfortable enough to require pain medication. The solution is left on your skin for several minutes. If your doctor uses glycolic acid, a chemical that penetrates more readily than other AHAs, it may be rinsed thoroughly with saline solution to neutralize its action and prevent harm to the skin. The other AHAs do not require rinsing. Finally, moisturizing cream is applied to your face.

Medium Peel

Like a light peel, a medium peel is performed in your physician's office. Your skin is cleansed and your doctor applies the solution to your face with a surgical sponge or cotton swab; this usually takes about ten to fifteen minutes. In about 45 seconds the chemical solution will cause your skin to turn a white, frosty color temporarily. This reaction is caused by the solution removing the surface skin cells.

Finally, you may sit under a fan for a while to help cool the burn. The burning sensation is stronger with a medium peel, so your doctor may suggest taking a mild sedative and ibuprofen beforehand.

Modified Deep Peel

A modified deep peel is usually done with twilight anesthesia in an accredited surgical facility. Even though the procedure carries less risk than the traditional deep

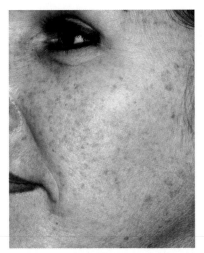
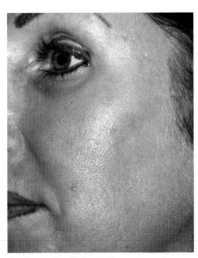
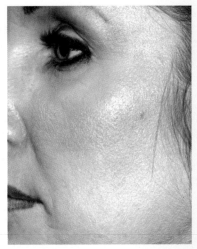

Before modified deep chemical peel.

One week after peel.

Four weeks after modified deep chemical peel.

peels, the patient's heart is monitored throughout the procedure; if too much phenol penetrates too deeply and enters the blood stream, it could cause heart rhythm disturbances.

Once you are asleep or comfortably dozing, your skin is cleansed and a solvent is used to remove surface oil to enable the solution to penetrate evenly. The peel solution is applied with applicator sticks, focusing on the areas with the most damage. A lighter application is applied to the other areas, taking care to blend the areas and feather the edges to prevent lines of demarcation. The entire procedure takes from 15 to 30 minutes.

Once the procedure is over, your doctor will cover your face with an emollient cream or petroleum jelly. The cream seals the skin, retaining moisture and preventing scab formation and scarring. When you awaken, the sensation is similar to a serious sunburn, easily relieved with pain medication. After you rest for an hour or two in the recovery area, you'll be ready to go home with your driver.

After Your Peel

Light Peel

For the next few days after a light peel your skin is likely to be somewhat pink and you may notice some mild dryness or flakiness. All these effects are easily camouflaged with light makeup, and soon you'll be aware only that your skin is fresher and smoother and that you're looking more rested than usual.

The flaking and dryness that follow an AHA peel are temporary and easily soothed with rich moisturizers and generous daily applications of a good, high-SPF sunscreen. Beyond that, there's no change in your daily skin routine; you can wear no makeup or as much as you wish.

Medium Peel

After a medium peel your skin will turn red, darken, peel, and in some cases may (or may not) develop some soft scabbed areas—better described as soft crusts—during the next several days. Crusting will depend on your skin condition and response to the treatment. The areas that received the greatest penetration of acid will be more likely to crust over.

You'll probably not want to go out. It usually takes up to two weeks to feel presentable again, although with makeup, you may feel comfortable after a week. Your skin color will gradually fade from red to a light pink. Once your new skin emerges, most of your fine wrinkles and blotches will have disappeared.

You shouldn't experience much discomfort, but if you do, ask your doctor for pain medication. Take the medication as needed over the next few days.

Avoid scratching or picking at your face and any crusts that may develop. Cleanse gently using the products your doctor provides for you to take home. Washing with water may be too drying, and your doctor will want you to protect your skin with appropriate cleansers and ointments. Avoid the sun completely for as long as possible, and once you do go out, never skip your full-spectrum sunblock.

Modified Deep Peel

The good news is that a modified deep peel produces remarkable results. The bad news? You'll look a whole lot worse before you look better. After the peel, your face will be very swollen for a day or so. During the first week, the swelling will be followed by peeling like that from a severe sunburn. Parts of your face will ooze.

Many patients report that while they don't have a lot of pain after this peel, they do feel a burning sensation for the first six to eight hours. Keeping the entire face moist with prescribed creams will prevent pain. Your doctor will prescribe mild pain medication, which you may wish to use, depending on how you're feeling.

You may find it uncomfortable to move your face. So you may not feel like talking for the first few days, and you may be more comfortable eating soft foods and drinking liquids, which require less chewing.

If you had any crusting, most of it will usually be gone after six to eight days. Your face will be very red, but you can begin to cover the redness with makeup. About a month after the procedure, your new skin will feel rough or even finely wrinkled. This will smooth out over the next six to eight weeks, and the redness will fade to baby-skin pink. The risk of permanent change in pigmentation is less with a modified deep peel than with the original deep peel. Your new skin is likely to be somewhat lighter, though a darker shade is also possible. If your entire face was peeled, any overall color change is less likely to be noticeable.

During the first five to ten days after your peel, you will need to keep the peel area covered with emollient cream or petroleum jelly, prescribed by your doctor. The peeled area must remain moist at all times until the oozing stops. Keeping the skin moist will prevent the skin from drying or crusting, which will create scarring. Also, avoid scarring by not picking or scratching your face as it heals.

When choosing a facial plastic surgeon, a patient should consider the doctor's training, specialization, experience, and results. He or she should invite you to speak with other patients. Listen to your "gut" feeling about the rapport you have with the surgeon.

— Dr. Jon Mendelsohn

To cleanse your face, gently use your fingertips and cool water. Pat your face dry with a clean towel and apply the cream your doctor has ordered. You'll need to continue this washing and moisturizing for seven to ten days. Your doctor will tell you when it's safe to wear makeup again and what cleansers and cosmetics to use.

Sleep on your back and use extra pillows until the swelling subsides. Keeping your head elevated will encourage the dissipation of the excess fluids that have collected in the tissue of your face.

For at least two months, postpone sports and recreation that expose you to the sun, ease slowly back into your exercise routine, and plan on wearing sunscreen forever. For example, use a large marble-sized dollop for your face and three marble-sized dollops for your neck and upper chest. Wait 30 minutes after applying it before you go out.

How Long Will Results Last?

Some people elect to repeat light peels every few weeks, but most doctors advise two- to three-month intervals. If light peels are done too often, they will dry the skin, and dryness promotes wrinkles. The exception to having a light peel every few weeks may be using a very light glycolic acid solution that is applied weekly for about six weeks, for the cumulative effect of a light peel.

Medium and deep peels last much longer. Although you might repeat a medium peel after one year if you have still not obtained the results you were aiming for, in most cases and with proper skin care, you're more likely to wait for years. Since modified deep peels remove the entire top layer of your facial skin, they produce permanent changes and a completely new skin surface.

Potential Risks

There are few risks with a light peel, other than possible lingering dryness. If you have had cold sores recently, a few weeks of antibiotic use beforehand is advisable.

If the herpes simplex virus that triggers cold sores is currently active in your skin, the peel could trigger a new outbreak with a risk of infection and scarring.

With medium peels there is some risk of permanent scarring, pigmentation change, uneven texture, or demarcation lines. These are uncommon complications when you're in the hands of a highly experienced professional. Infection is also a potential risk. Closely following your doctor's aftercare instructions greatly reduces your risk of infection. Your doctor may also prescribe an antibiotic.

As mentioned earlier, modified deep peels can cause heart rhythm disturbances and lasting kidney damage in some people if too much phenol enters the skin. This risk is reduced when less phenol is used, and careful medical monitoring during the procedure should prevent problems. As with medium peels, permanent skin pigmentation changes, in which skin color becomes paler or uneven, are also possible.

Surgical skin resurfacing may give your face that youthful glow you're hoping for— if you have fair or light-brown skin. Deep peels, laser resurfacing, and dermabrasion are not recommended for types IV, V, or VI on the Fitzpatrick Classification skin type chart. If you fall into one of these categories, talk to your facial plastic surgeon about alternatives, perhaps including microdermabrasion or light to medium chemical peels.

Fitzpatrick Classification of Skin Type		
Skin Type	Description	Reaction to Sun
I	Pale white or freckled	Always burns, never tans
II	White	Always burns easily, tans minimally
III	White to light brown	Burns moderately, tans uniformly
IV	Moderate brown	Burns minimally, always tans well
V	Dark brown	Rarely burns, tans profusely
VI	Very dark brown to black	Never burns

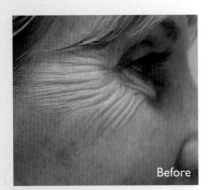

Before

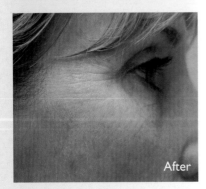

After

Two weeks after botox injections.

Nonsurgical Procedures

No doubt you've heard about the many newer, nonsurgical procedures that are available for rejuvenating the skin. Many of these procedures are considered "lunch hour" procedures—you can have them done over your lunch hour and return to work. These procedures are among the most popular cosmetic procedures performed today.

Botox

Botox™ and *Myobloc™* are brand names for diluted *botulinum toxin* used in extremely small doses to treat forehead lines, frown lines, smile lines, crow's feet, smoker's lines, marionette lines, chin dents, neck bands, and sagging brows. Injections of Botox smooth the skin, reducing fine lines and superficial wrinkles by preventing the facial movement that causes them.

A Botox treatment is an outpatient procedure that takes five to ten minutes. No anesthesia is needed; discomfort, if any, lasts just a few seconds. Using a tiny needle, the doctor injects small amounts of Botox, one to three injections per muscle, into the muscle surrounding the wrinkle being treated. It may take a few weeks for you to see the benefits, which peak at one to two weeks. Repeat procedures every three or four months are recommended.

You'll want to delay Botox if you are pregnant or nursing or if you're taking certain medications, including some antibiotics, anti-inflammatory drugs, aspirin, and certain vitamins and herbs. (Your doctor will give you a complete list.)

After a Botox treatment, avoid rubbing the area for 24 hours. Some doctors tell their Botox patients to remain upright for several hours and to avoid alcohol for a few days.

Microdermabrasion

Microdermabrasion involves your doctor or a technician using a device, about the size of a ballpoint pen, that showers your face with fine granules or crystals to

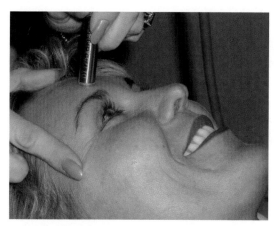

Microdermabrasion uses sterile crystals to exfoliate the top layer of skin and simultaneously vacuums the dead skin cells.

remove dead skin cells. Some people refer to it as a miniature version of sandblasting. The result is a healthy glow, with reduction of fine lines, age spots, acne scars, thickened skin, blemishes, and large pores. In addition, the procedure stimulates the production of skin cells and collagen. The results of microdermabrasion may be apparent for several months. Many doctors recommend five or more initial treatments spaced about two weeks apart plus maintenance treatments every three months or so.

Microdermabrasion is not intended for major acne scarring, tattoos, or deep wrinkles. Ask your doctor about other procedures if these are your concerns. Delay having microdermabrasion if you have active sores or a rash on your face or if you have recently had an oral herpes outbreak. Avoid using exfoliating lotions (such as AHA and Retin-A) and scrubs for three days before and after treatment.

It takes 20 to 30 minutes to treat the full face. No anesthesia is required. You'll feel nothing more than a slight burning—comparable to sunburn or windburn—during and for a few hours after the procedure. Don't wear foundation for a day or so, and stay out of the sun for at least a week.

Beware of nonsterile conditions and inexperienced, unskilled microdermabrasion technicians. Microdermabrasion is safe if performed properly in a sterile environment. Otherwise, serious complications, including scarring and infection, are possible.

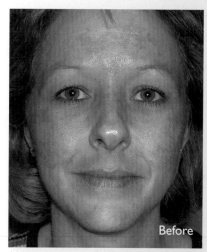

Before

Mottled pigmentation and rough skin.

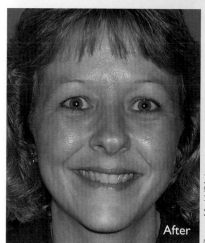

After

After seven weekly microdermabrasion treatments, skin is smoother and skin tone is even.

Derma Med USA, Inc.

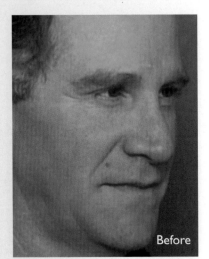

Low eyebrows—before thermage of forehead.

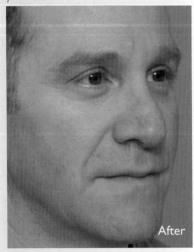

Thermage has tightened underlying collagen, resulting in a lifting of the eyebrows.

Thermoplasty

With thermoplasty—also known as *ThermaCool TC™*, *Thermage™*, or *ThermaLift™* —your doctor uses a radiofrequency-generating device to apply intense heat to the underlying skin, while bursts of cryogen spray cool the outer skin layers. The process can cause immediate tightening of the collagen network, which may tighten and lift your skin. It also stimulates the gradual formation of new collagen, which may thicken the skin to reduce wrinkling and tighten pores anywhere on the face.

Though some patients have reported good results with one treatment, some doctors recommend an initial series of treatments plus touchups as needed. Full benefits will appear three to six months after treatment and may last several years. Occasionally these results are dramatic; more commonly, the change is much less apparent and will not provide the improvement possible with surgical procedures.

You'll probably be given a sedative and local anesthesia before your thermoplasty treatment, so arrange for someone to drive you to and from the doctor's office.

Afterward you may feel as though you're sunburned. About half of thermoplasty patients have slight swelling for four to five days. Temporary bruising and numbness are unusual. Your doctor will let you know when you can resume your normal activities.

IPL Photorejuvenation

Intense pulsed light, or *IPL photorejuvenation*, is a new, noninvasive technique that can even out skin color and texture. Effective on brown and red spots, the procedure can improve hyperpigmentation, blemishes, rosacea, spider veins, age spots, sun damage, freckles, enlarged pores, and birthmarks. It may also minimize fine lines and wrinkles, giving you smoother, younger-looking skin.

IPL photorejuvenation does not use lasers; instead it delivers ultraviolet and other types of light in pulses that have been compared to a camera flash. Brown and red spots absorb more of this pulsed light than does surrounding tissue—enough to destroy the darker cells, which will eventually fade away. IPL also stimulates collagen production, which works to firm and smooth your skin.

Your doctor will probably tell you to stay out of the sun for several weeks before and after your IPL treatment. Tanning may cause your skin to absorb too much light during the treatment. Sun exposure afterward can be especially harmful to your newly treated skin.

If you have a history of oral herpes (cold sores or fever blisters), your doctor may prescribe an antiviral drug for you to take before treatment to guard against a breakout. Be sure to tell your doctor what medications you're taking. You may need to discontinue certain medications before treatment. If you are pregnant, postpone IPL photorejuvenation until after your baby arrives.

Treatments are usually short, lasting 15 to 45 minutes. A cold gel will be applied to the treatment area, and your doctor may also use a topical anesthetic, though most patients report feeling no discomfort or only a slight sting without anesthesia. You'll wear protective goggles or eye shields to prevent eye damage as the doctor or assistant delivers the pulsed light with a handheld IPL device.

Patients generally have five to six treatments, each separated by about three weeks. The results can be very long lasting, though some doctors recommend that patients have one or two treatments per year after the initial series.

Expect nothing more than slight redness or swelling that will last only a day or two. Many patients go right back to work after their treatments. Occasionally, a patient will have bruises or blisters.

Questions to Ask Your Doctor

- What are your medical credentials?
- What type of peel is appropriate for me?
- How quickly will I recover?
- How should I care for my skin before and after the peel?
- Should I stop taking my usual medications or supplements?
- Do I have any condition that would make me a poor candidate for laser treatment?
- If I have a series of nonablative laser treatments, how far apart should they be?
- How many initial treatments would you recommend for me?
- Is laser therapy likely to achieve the improvement I'm looking for?

CHAPTER 14

SCAR REVISION

14

SCAR REVISION

cars come in all shapes and sizes. They can be flat or raised, darker or lighter than your own skin, smooth or puckered. Many scars—such as those from burns, cuts, and scrapes—can result from an infection or inflammation. Of course, scars can also come from surgery. Whatever the cause, scars often cause us embarrassment when they appear on our faces. However, today's surgical techniques make it possible to revise scars, making them much less noticeable.

What Causes Scars?

Scars are actually nature's way of protecting you. When skin is damaged or lost, your body's natural response is to form collagen, which supports healing, replaces the injured skin, and protects the area from infection and outside irritants.

The characteristics of a scar depend on many factors, including:

- The size, direction, and depth of the original injury

- Its location on your body and the blood supply to that area

- Your age at the time of injury

- Your skin characteristics, including thickness and color

- Your overall health and nutrition.

Types of Scars

Contracture Scars

Contracture scars develop after a large area of skin is lost. This often results from burns. These scars are contracted, meaning they are tight or puckered, because they cover a smaller area than the original skin, sometimes pulling on nearby muscles and tendons.

Keloid Scars

Keloids occur when collagen formation, which occurs naturally after an injury, continues after the wound has healed, causing these scars to spill out of the boundaries of the wound. These scars may be thick, puckered, or "ropey" and tend to be red or darker than the surrounding skin. Some keloids grow to resemble tumors. The scars may itch or cause a burning sensation.

Though keloids can occur anywhere on the body, they tend to form on the chest, the shoulders, the back, or the earlobes, usually after ear piercing. Keloids rarely occur on the face but may occur on the neck or jawline. More common in people with thick or dark skin, a keloid can develop a year or more after the original injury. Keloids are so stubborn that they often return despite a surgeon's best efforts to remove them.

Hypertrophic Scars

Hypertrophic scars are overdeveloped scars that occur most often when a wound's healing is delayed, for example by infection or reinjury. Though hypertrophic scars may be thick, red, and ropey like keloids, they differ from keloids in that they stay within the boundaries of the original wound. Hypertrophic scars may improve on their own or with steroid applications or injections. When they are removed surgically, they usually don't come back as keloids often do.

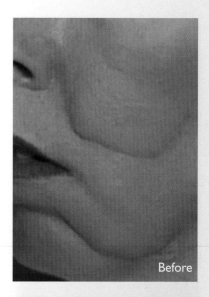

Before

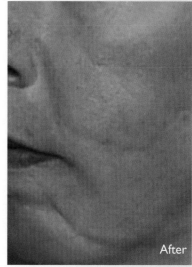

After

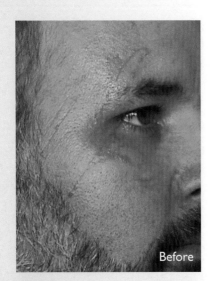

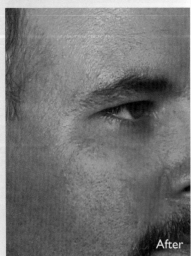

Scar revision with laser skin resurfacing.

Hypopigmented Scars

Hypopigmented scars are whitish, silverish or pale in color due to a lack of the skin pigment melanin, the substance that gives color to skin. These scars result when pigment-producing cells are damaged by broken blood vessels and inflammation. Sometimes scars that are lighter than the surrounding skin are treated with *micropigmentation*—basically tattooing the scar tissue. If you choose this method, find a micropigmentation technician who is skilled and experienced in scar camouflage. Ask your plastic surgeon for a recommendation.

You might also ask your surgeon to recommend a licensed cosmetologist. Someone who is experienced in camouflaging all kinds of scars can be a tremendous help to you both before and after your scar revision procedure.

Scars are permanent, though many fade, practically becoming invisible with time. Qualified plastic surgeons experienced in scar revision do an excellent job of camouflaging facial scars using a variety of techniques.

Are You a Candidate?

The best candidates for scar revision surgery understand these benefits and limitations and are willing to follow the surgeon's instructions before and after the procedure. Some doctors believe the best time for scar revision surgery is a few months after a scar develops, when it is fairly new. Others prefer to wait a year or more until the scar is completely healed and has thinned and lightened.

Your plastic surgeon will recommend the scar revision technique that will best improve your appearance. A series of treatments may be needed, and some scars, especially keloids, can recur, as mentioned above. Although the proper treatment can make your scar less obvious and greatly improve its appearance, no scar can be completely removed.

Scar Revision Therapies

Steroids

The initial treatment for keloid and hypertrophic scars is usually cortical steroid injections. When injected into scar tissue, these steroids can reduce itching, burning, and redness and may break down collagen, shrinking the scar as well. Topical steroids may be applied during surgery and for up to two years afterward.

Also, applications of *silicone sheeting*, which are rubber-like bandages containing silicone, may lighten and flatten scars over a period of several weeks; they may also prevent keloids from developing. How does the silicone work? It is believed that static electricity from the silicone helps align collagen fibers in the scar. It is also possible that the silicone traps moisture, which can help scars fade.

Laser Treatments

To smooth rough or raised scars, your surgeon may use a series of laser treatments over a six- to eight-week period. High-intensity laser light can flatten scars and change their color to blend better with surrounding skin. There is usually some bruising immediately after the treatment. A mild degree of pigment change occurs in approximately 20 percent of cases, but is usually temporary.

Cryotherapy

Cryotherapy involves the scar being frozen off by a medication. Liquid nitrogen is applied or sprayed onto the scar, causing the scar to blister. With repeated treatments, the scar usually flattens. This technique carries the risk of depigmentation around the scar area.

Pressure Therapy

Pressure therapy involves a type of pressure appliance worn over the area of the scar. These may be worn day and night for up to four to six months.

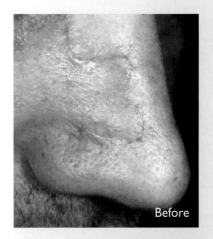
Before

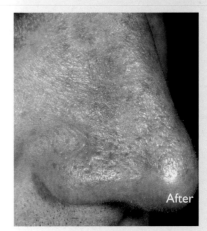
After

The laser eliminated the scar by resurfacing the top layer of skin.

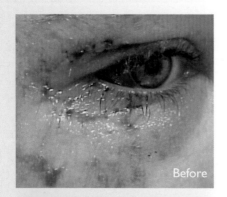
Before

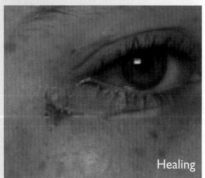
Healing

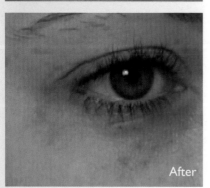
After

Scar Revision Surgery

Treatment for scars may also involve surgery to remove the scar tissue and replace it with healthy skin. This skin may be in the form of a *skin graft*, which is taken from another area of the body. When transplanted, these thin layers of healthy skin interact with the surrounding tissues to form a new blood supply.

A second option is for the skin to come from a flap, which is adjacent skin and underlying tissue that is lifted and moved. Skin flaps bring their blood supply to the new site, since not only healthy skin but also its underlying fat, nerves, blood vessels, and muscle are moved from the donor site to the scarred site. Skin flaps and grafts are often performed in an ambulatory surgery center or in a hospital under general anesthesia. However, it is not uncommon for smaller flaps and grafts to be performed in a surgeon's office suite.

The surgeon may combine surgical removal with steroid applications, and patients may have to wear a pressure dressing for many months after the scar removal procedure.

W-plasty and Z-plasty

Your surgeon can camouflage a straight scar by removing the scar and making new incisions that are harder to see. The surgeon may make a zigzag incision, which is referred to as *W-plasty* or *zigzag plasty*. Or your surgeon may make a new incision using a Z shape, known as *Z-plasty*. These approaches change the direction of the scar, interrupt the scar line, and lengthen the scar. As a result, the irregular lines are harder for the eye to follow and are less obvious than straight lines.

After Your Scar Revision Surgery

As you recover, your scar may look worse before it looks better. It can take a year or longer for the benefits to be fully apparent. Your doctor might have you wear a compression bandage; the length of time you may need to wear it depends on the type of scar. You should stay out of the sun and away from tanning beds for up to a year.

Side Effects, Risks, and Complications

Short-term bruising, redness, swelling, and slight bleeding from the incision are common after scar revision surgery. Scars are unpredictable, and there's a small chance your scar won't be improved by surgery or that some scarring, especially keloids, may recur.

Questions to Ask the Surgeon

- What type of scar do I have?
- Which scar revision procedure can make my scar less obvious?
- Is the scar likely to come back after surgery?
- What can I do to promote healing and a good outcome?
- How long will the results of my surgery last?

CHAPTER 15

FOLLOW-UP SKIN CARE

FOLLOW-UP SKIN CARE

icture yourself looking fantastic with balanced facial features and smooth, radiant skin. Facial cosmetic surgery can help make that vision a reality, but follow-up skin care is important to help maintain the results of your surgery. Doing everything you can to make your new look last means taking tender care of yourself all over.

The very best thing you can do for your skin is to keep yourself in glowing good health. Beware of your skin's worst enemies: stress, lack of sleep, smoking and environmental pollutants, inadequate water intake, excess sunshine, a sedentary lifestyle, and a poor diet. The following fundamentals will help you maintain healthy skin after your cosmetic procedure.

- Be good to yourself. You can't avoid stress altogether, but you can see to it that your needs for quiet time, recreation, and stress reducers are met.

- Get enough sleep—seven to eight hours every night. Restful sleep gives your cells a chance to repair themselves.

- Don't smoke. It wreaks havoc on your skin and other organs as well.

- Remember that sweat is friend and enemy alike; it leaches toxins out of your skin, but essential salts and minerals are lost, too. Don't leave sweat on your skin any longer than necessary; the toxins can clog your pores.

- Exercise regularly to increase blood flow, which supplies oxygen and nutrients to your skin and other organs.

- Eat those veggies! Be sure you're getting enough fiber, protein, and other nutrients needed by your skin and the rest of you. Avoid simple sugars, greasy snacks, and highly processed foods.

Good Skin Care

Pampering your skin can be a relaxing ritual, but even if you don't have time to indulge yourself, do follow the four basic steps of facial skin care: cleanse, exfoliate, moisturize, and protect.

Normal Skin

Complete facial cleansing is most important at night when you're washing off the residue of the day—bacteria, sweat, pollutants, and especially makeup, whose pigments can irritate the skin and clog the pores. Remove every trace of makeup before you go to bed, including mascara, especially if it's waterproof. The flecks can work their way into your eyes while you sleep. Here are tips for cleansing:

- If you use the mildest cleanser that will do the job and rinse thoroughly, you shouldn't need a toner to remove drying residues.

- Avoid scented cleansers and moisturizers.

- Cleanse the skin on your neck, too.

- Keep your hands away from your face to avoid transmitting oils and bacteria.

Dry Skin

Use a cleansing cream or lotion or a very mild soap with water. Antibacterial and deodorant soaps are too harsh for the face. If the product lathers easily, it may be too drying.

Wash your face and neck at night when your skin has time to replenish the oils that washing strips away. Rinse thoroughly with lukewarm water. Pat your skin dry—don't rub—with a clean towel. In the morning, just rinse with lukewarm water and pat dry. Don't use astringents, clarifying lotions, or toners unless they are labeled "moisturizing." Avoid those containing alcohol, witch hazel, and other drying ingredients.

Avoid steam baths and saunas; excessive sweating takes natural moisture out of your skin. In winter, turn down the thermostat. Heat from your furnace dries out the air, as does air conditioning in summer, especially in dry climates. Humidifiers and well-watered houseplants can put needed moisture back into the air.

Take warm, not hot, baths and showers, and keep them short.

Oily Skin

If your skin is oily, your instincts say, "Dry it out." Your instincts may be right, but be careful how you do it. Wash and rinse your face with warm or hot water no more than twice a day. You can actually overcleanse and overdry your skin by washing it too often and using harsh products or super-hot water. The important thing is to keep your skin clean without stripping away its natural protection.

Use a mild, oil-free cleanser. Antibacterial and deodorant soaps are too drying for even the oiliest facial skin. Your face shouldn't feel tight or dry after washing.

Look for products labeled *noncomedogenic*, meaning they won't clog your pores. If your face feels oily between washings, use astringent pads.

Dead skin cells clog pores and allow moisture to escape, so use an *exfoliant* formulated for oily skin three or four times a week. Try a mild facial scrub with small granules, or use a soft, clean face brush or sponge. The body scrubs with shell or seed granules are too harsh for the face.

You might not need to moisturize, but if you do, read product labels. Ingredients to look for include witch hazel, beeswax, some vegetable oils (corn or safflower), sodium lauryl sulfate, octyl palmitate, AHA, and BHA. Ingredients to avoid include most other oils (petrolatum, mineral oil, coconut oil, and olive oil for example), lanolin, cold cream, cocoa butter, isopropyl myristate, and oleic acid.

Choose water-based, oil-free makeup and make sure you remove it thoroughly before going to bed.

Exfoliating Your Skin

A skin exfoliant removes dead cells on the skin's surface, revealing fresher skin underneath and preventing clogged pores. You can exfoliate by mechanical means—with a cleanser containing small granules or with a soft brush—or chemically, with products such as hydroxy acids and *tretinoin*.

Don't combine exfoliants or use more than one exfoliating product unless your facial plastic surgeon or dermatologist tells you to do so; too much can damage

---

Makeup Tips

- When you're shopping for makeup, don't use testers on your face.

- Buy from trusted manufacturers.

- Don't share makeup with anyone. You're not being selfish; you're being safe.

- Wash makeup sponges, powder puffs, and other applicators every other day with antibacterial soap.

- Discard any cosmetics that change color or develop an odor.

- If you develop a skin infection on your face or in your eye, throw away all the makeup you've been using on the infected area.

your skin. Exfoliating three to four times a week may be adequate.

Using Alpha Hydroxy Acid and Beta Hydroxy Acid

Alpha hydroxy acid (AHA) is commonly used as an exfoliant. AHA lifts away dead cells from the skin's surface and may also stimulate new collagen and elastin growth below the skin's surface. When Cleopatra, Queen of the Nile, bathed in sour milk more than two thousand years ago, she was soaking her skin in *lactic acid,* a form of AHA. *Glycolic acid* (from sugar cane) and lactic acid are favored in skin products for their ability to penetrate the epidermis. The U.S. Food and Drug Administration (FDA) considers AHA safe for consumer use at a concentration of 10 percent or lower and a pH of 3.5 or higher. Skin care experts recommend an AHA concentration between 5 and 10 percent with a pH between 3.5 and 4. After six months of using such a product, you could see improvement in wrinkles, rough skin, and uneven pigmentation.

Beta hydroxy acid (BHA) is often listed on ingredient labels as *salicylic acid*—the active ingredient in aspirin. Whereas AHA is water-soluble, BHA is *lipid-soluble*—able to dissolve in oil—making it a better choice for oily skin. BHA can actually penetrate the *sebum*, a natural skin oil in pores, and slough off the accumulated dead skin cells, unclogging the pores and refreshing the skin. After six months of regular use, BHA can help correct fine lines and wrinkles and make your skin smoother, as well as reducing blackheads, whiteheads, and other oily blemishes. It works best in formulations of 1 to 2 percent at a pH of 3 to 4.

Both AHA and BHA can irritate sensitive skin. Concentrations higher than the FDA recommendations can cause burns and should be used only if a doctor prescribes them. The hydroxy acids make your skin more sun-sensitive by about 50 percent, so you must use sun protection faithfully. AHA and BHA also may cause pigment changes, especially on dark skin. Some experts recommend you use AHA or BHA in only one skin care product, preferably a moisturizer. Hydroxy acids in cleansers aren't on your skin long enough to accomplish anything.

Using Tretinoin—Retin-A and Renova

These topical skin preparations, derivations of vitamin A, exfoliate the skin, stimulate collagen production, and even out skin pigments. They may also prevent development of precancerous growths such as actinic keratoses.

Though Retin-A was approved for acne treatment in 1971 and Renova for skin damage in 1996, the major difference is Renova's *emollient*, a soothing and smoothing base that may prevent irritation better than Retin-A. Neither Renova nor Retin-A is a moisturizer, however, and you'll need to use moisturizer if your skin is dry, as well as a sunscreen over either product.

Tretinoin always makes your skin sun sensitive, and you can get a blistering burn—even in the shade—if you don't protect your skin. If you use tretinoin only at night and wash it off in the morning before you go outside, you'll still need sun protection.

You should not use tretinoin if you are pregnant or planning to become pregnant. In addition to sun sensitivity, both Renova and Retin-A can cause redness, irritation, dryness, and peeling. If you have these symptoms, stop using tretinoin and call your doctor. You might need to use a lower concentration or switch to another product, such as AHA.

Moisturizing Your Skin

Your moisturizer won't add moisture to your skin. What it will do is prevent water loss by covering your face with a layer of oil, or by attracting your body's moisture to the upper skin layers, or both. These products should be applied to the face and neck.

Different skin types have different needs. Since you most likely use moisturizer every day, become a savvy consumer—read and understand ingredient labels.

Types of Moisturizers

The main difference among ointments, creams, and lotions is the amount of oil they contain. Ointments have the most oil. Lotions have the least. All moisturizers contain emollients plus occlusives or humectants, or both.

Occlusives—ingredients that physically block moisture loss—include petrolatum, mineral and vegetable oils, lanolin, zinc oxide, and silicone. *Humectants*—substances that attract and retain moisture—contain no oil. Glycerin, sorbitol, urea, hydroxy acids, hyaluronic acid, propylene glycol, and sugars may act as humectants in moisturizers. Products containing hydroxy acids should either contain sunscreen or instruct the user to use sun protection.

Lubricating *emollients* smooth the face by filling spaces within the skin. Common examples are petrolatum, mineral oil, fatty acids, plant oils, shea butter, cocoa butter, animal oils, (including lanolin and emu), cholesterol, triglycerides, palmitates, myristates, stearates, and ceramides. If you read ingredient labels, you'll see these names often.

Moisturizers may contain other ingredients as well:

- *Antioxidants* such as selenium, vitamin A (retinyl palmitate, retinol), vitamin C (ascorbic acid, ascorbyl palmitate), vitamin D, vitamin E (a-Tocopherol), coenzyme Q-10, alpha lipoic acid, green tea, grape extract, and others. Antioxidants taken as food supplements may protect the body's cells against free radicals—a very reactive, unstable form of oxygen that can cause tissue damage and illness, including cancer. Recent studies suggest that many *topical* antioxidants—those applied to the skin—can penetrate the top skin layer to fight free radicals.

- *Rejuvenators*—the proteins collagen, elastin, and keratin—may add more to a product's cost than they're worth. Though all three proteins are building blocks of healthy skin, when applied on top of the skin they probably have little effect since the large protein molecules can't penetrate very deeply.

It may be helpful to understand how some of these ingredients may affect your skin. *Mineral oil* and *petrolatum* do an excellent job of locking in moisture, but products in which mineral oil or petrolatum is the main ingredient can make your skin feel greasy or sticky, clog pores, and trap perspiration. Silicones and plant oils are often used as alternatives.

Vitamins in moisturizers can promote healing. That's been proven with vitamin C. Vitamin E's healing properties are in dispute, though an entire generation of moms claim there's nothing like the gooey contents of a vitamin E capsule for protecting and healing small cuts and scrapes.

Essential fatty acids (EFAs) support skin moisture and elasticity. You can take them orally or as ingredients in skin products. They are found in many plant and animal oils, including fish, emu, flaxseed, borage, primrose, vegetable, coconut, and grapeseed. You may see EFAs on cosmetic labels as linoleic or alpha-linoleic acid.

It may sound strange to learn that *propylene glycol* is the main ingredient in car antifreeze. In lower concentrations it's also a humectant that helps keep your skin, as well as your moisturizer, from drying out. It's highly toxic if you drink it, but the small amount in cosmetics is believed to be harmless when absorbed through the skin.

Parabens, an ingredient that is usually prefaced by *methyl-, propyl-, ethyl-,* or *butyl-,* are the most common cosmetic preservatives used in the United States. They are generally considered safe for external use, though a recent study has linked breast cancer to parabens in underarm deodorants.

Special Care for Sensitive Skin

If your skin is sensitive, you may be drawn to products labeled "hypoallergenic." The list of ingredients identified as potential irritants or toxins that can be absorbed through the skin is long, but the FDA and the Cosmetic, Toiletry, and Fragrance Association consider FDA-approved substances safe as used in cosmetics.

Though hypoallergenic products may indeed contain fewer ingredients likely to cause sensitivity or allergic reactions, the FDA requires allergy testing of all products sold as cosmetics. A partial list of ingredients that can irritate the skin or cause allergic reactions includes lanolin (which is derived from sheep's wool), glycerin, sunscreens, plant extracts, urea, lactic acid, fragrance, parabens, formaldehyde, even aloe vera.

Oddly enough, aloe vera is also considered an anti-irritant. Other anti-irritants include allantoin, licorice root, glycyrrhetinic acid, green tea, vitamin C, chamomile extract, and willow bark. Aloe vera in moisturizers might not be concentrated enough to do much good. Look for pure aloe vera gel and mix it with your moisturizer or use it separately.

Avoiding Sun Damage

You may have thought that simply getting older is the reason your face ages. Certainly, chronological aging leaves its mark on your face. But the truth is that the single most powerful force working to alter your smooth, healthy skin is sun exposure. It's estimated that 80 percent of aging of the skin is caused by the sun. Sun causes photoaging or premature wrinkling as well as blotches, broken blood vessels, dryness, and thinning.

The ultraviolet (UV) rays do the damage, and there are two types. UV-A rays gradually and invisibly weaken collagen, the protein-rich supporting layer that keeps your skin firm, supple, and wrinkle-resistant. UV-B rays cause burning and tanning and set the stage for skin cancer.

Sunlamps and tanning beds also damage the skin, and many doctors believe that tanning pills are harmful as well. They may cause yellow deposits to form in the retina. Indoor tanning lotions are the safest way to brown your skin, and today's products won't turn you orange as early products did, but they don't usually contain sunscreen so you'll have to layer some on over the tanner.

Using Sunscreen

Sunscreens work by reflecting or absorbing ultraviolet rays, or both. A sunscreen's SPF, or *sun protection factor*, indicates how long it will take you to get sunburned if you're using the product. If you normally burn after half an hour in the sun, it would take ten times longer (five hours) to burn when you're wearing sunscreen that has an SPF of 10.

Ingredients that reflect UVR are called sunscreens or sunblocks and include zinc oxide and titanium dioxide; these rarely if ever cause allergic reactions. Chemicals that absorb UVR include PABA, Parsol 1789™, and cinnamates. Some people are allergic or sensitive to these products, as well as salicylates, oxybenzone, lanolin, fragrances, and other sunscreen ingredients. If you develop itching, a rash, blisters, or hives after using sunscreen, ask your doctor to recommend a product less likely to bring on sensitivity or allergic reactions.

Look for *broad-spectrum sunscreens*. The SPF on the label refers to UV-B protection, but the ingredients that prevent tanning offer some protection against UV-A radiation as well. Sunscreens offering the best UV-A protection contain either opaque ingredients (titanium dioxide or zinc oxide) or Parsol 1789, which may be listed as avobenzone or dibenzoylmethane. Newer transparent sunscreens may contain opaque ingredients in powder form. Look for the words "microfine" or "Z-COTE" on the label.

Get in the habit of applying at least one full ounce of sunscreen to your entire body every day. Most doctors recommend sunscreens with an SPF of 15 or higher. An SPF 10 blocks about 85 percent of UVR, SPF 15 about 95 percent, and SPF 30 about 97 percent.

Apply your sunscreen indoors and stay out of the sun for another 20 to 30 minutes. Even if it's labeled water resistant, reapply the sunscreen when you've been sweating and after you've been in the water.

Sunscreen does keep your skin from absorbing the vitamin D in sunlight, so take a vitamin D supplement or make sure you're getting enough of this essential nutrient in your diet.

Protect your delicate eye area with a sunscreen labeled safe for eyes, and always wear a lip product with an SPF of at least 15.

When the sun's rays start burning your skin, it fights back by producing melanin, the pigment that tans and thus protects the skin. But a tan is weak protection compared to sunscreen or clothing. Even a dark tan has an SPF of only about 4.

Wear Protective Clothing

Clothing offers some protection against the sun's rays; however, UVR can easily penetrate some fabrics, including swimsuits, especially when they're wet. A white T-shirt has an SPF of 6. To stay both cool and protected, wear lightweight, dark-colored, tightly woven, loose fitting clothes that cover your arms and legs.

Wear a sun-protective hat, preferably one with a full brim that protects your ears and the back of your neck as well as your eyes and face. You'll still need sunscreen. A 7-centimeter hat brim provides an estimated SPF of 20 on your forehead but as little as SPF 4 on your nose.

Good sunglasses prevent squinting, and the crow's feet that follow, and protect delicate eyelid skin from aging. Look for sunglasses that block 99 to 100 percent of the sun's rays and that wrap around to protect your eyes from the sides as well as the front.

Questions to Ask the Surgeon

- Would my skin be improved with prescription tretinoin, Retin-A or Renova?

- Are there high enough concentrations of AHA in over-the-counter products to benefit my skin?

- If I have an allergic reaction to an over-the-counter cosmetic, how will I know which ingredient caused it?

- Do you recommend a sunscreen for my geographical region?

- If I do get sunburn, what is the best way to treat it?

GLOSSARY

ablative laser: a laser capable of ablating (carrying away, removing) a layer of skin.

Accutane™: a drug derived from vitamin A and used to treat acne.

actinic keratosis: a flat, scaly skin lesion caused by sun damage and often precancerous.

Advanta™: a synthetic facial implant, a form of Gore-Tex, that is FDA-approved for the enhancement of facial folds, lines, and wrinkles.

AHA: see *alpha hydroxy acid.*

Alloderm™: the brand name for cadaveric skin (human skin from a dead body) that is specially processed and precut for implantation.

alopecia: hair loss.

alpha hydroxy acid (AHA): an exfoliant derived from sugar cane, milk, or citrus fruit; used in some chemical peels and skin products.

anabolic steroids: hormones and hormone-like substances derived from natural or synthetic testosterone.

anticoagulant: any of several substances that inhibit blood clot formation.

antioxidant: a chemical that attacks free radicals.

asymmetry: imbalance; being not the same on both sides.

auricle: the visible outer portion of the ear; a projecting structure of skin cartilage.

autologous: derived from one's own body.

beta hydroxy acid (BHA): an oil-soluble exfoliant used in some skin products to remove outer skin.

Bichat's fat pad: see *buccal fat pad.*

bioimplant: implants that function like a scaffold to be filled in slowly by your body's own collagen.

blepharoplasty: eyelid lift.

Botox™: an injectable, medical-grade, weakened form of Botulinum Toxin Type A.

Botulinum Toxin Type A: a neurotoxin that in weakened form causes temporary muscle paralysis; useful in medical applications and for smoothing and contouring the face.

bovine collagen: a connective tissue protein derived from cows and used in injectable form to help correct facial wrinkles.

broad-spectrum sunscreen: a skin protection product that screens both UV-A and UV-B rays.

browlift: cosmetic surgery to elevate the brows, soften lines, and correct heavy upper eyelids by removing, tightening, or repositioning tissues.

buccal fat pad: a small mass of fat under the skin in the middle part of the face.

butylparaben: see *parabens.*

carbolic acid: see *phenol.*

cheek lift: see *midface lift.*

chemical peel: a procedure in which chemicals are used to remove the skin's outer layers.

chin implantation: surgery to place solid implants into the chin.

chinplasty: see *chin implantation.*

chondritis: inflammation of cartilage.

collagen: a protein that supports the skin (and other soft tissues) and bones.

columella: the strip of tissue separating the nostrils.

composite facelift: a lift that tightens all facial layers down to the bone and has more long lasting results.

concha: the hollow, bowl-like portion of the outer ear next to the canal.

conjunctiva: a thin, moist membrane that lines the underside of the eyelid and the exposed part of the eyelids.

constricted ear: a condition in which the helix (outer rim of the ear) is tightened, hooded, or folded.

contracture: abnormal shortening of soft tissues; a scar covering a smaller area than the original skin, sometimes pulling on nearby muscles and tendons and restricting range of motion.

coronal incision: a large surgical cut that goes from ear to ear across the top of the head.

corrugator muscles: small, fan-shaped muscles that lie under the inner portions of the eyebrows; part of the network of muscles of facial expression.

cortical steroids, corticosteroids: natural or synthetic hormones used to control swelling and inflammation.

Croton oil: an oil, prepared from the seeds of the Croton Tiglium tree, used in some chemical peel solutions.

cryotherapy: the use of very cold or frozen products to reduce discomfort, limit progression of tissue edema, or break a cycle of muscle spasm.

cup ear: a type of constricted ear in which the helix folds down, the concha is enlarged, and the ear protrudes, making the ear look unusually small.

Cupid's bow: the double curve of the upper lip.

deep-plane facelift: a facelift performed at a deeper level, separating the muscle from the bone and lifting the muscle.

dermabrasion: a surgical procedure that uses a high-speed rotating brush to remove the upper layers of skin.

dermaplaning: a procedure that uses a handheld instrument, similar to a scalpel, to scrape dead cells from the skin surface.

dermis: the thickest of the skin layers, making up about 90 percent of the skin's thickness.

direct browlift: a type of forehead lift in which the skin just above the eyebrows is removed.

edema: swelling caused by the accumulation of fluid in body tissues.

EFAs: see *essential fatty acids.*

elastin: a protein that gives the skin elasticity, tone, and texture.

emollient: a substance that softens and smoothes the skin by preventing water loss.

endoscopic: relating to *endoscopy,* a procedure in which a doctor examines and sometimes manipulates structures inside the body through a lighted flexible tube called an *endoscope.*

endoscopic browlift: a browlift performed through a small incision and guided by a tiny TV camera.

epidermis: the skin's outer protective layers.

ePTFE: see *expanded polytetrafluoroethylene.*

essential fatty acids (EFAs): substances found in many plant and animal oils that support skin moisture and elasticity.

ethylparaben: see *parabens.*

exfoliant: a substance or device that removes dead cells from the skin's surface.

expanded polytetrafluoroethylene (ePTFE): a synthetic polymer derived from carbon and often used as an implant material.

extrusion: a condition of bulging or protruding.

eyelid retraction: a condition in which the lower lid becomes lax after surgery and may pull away from the eye.

facial plastic surgeon: a highly specialized medical doctor whose training is specific to diseases, defects, and cosmetic abnormalities of the face and neck.

fascia: strong connective membranes under the skin.

fat pad: see *buccal fat pad.*

filler implant: a synthetic or organic material introduced into a face or other body part for smoothing, augmenting, or firming.

filler injection: a procedure that smoothes facial irregularities by introducing a gel-like substance with a small needle.

forehead lift: see *browlift.*

free radical: a very reactive, unstable form of oxygen that can cause tissue damage and illness, including cancer.

frontalis muscle: a broad, flat muscle of facial expression spanning the forehead, functioning to raise the eyebrows.

general anesthesia: method used to stop pain from being felt during a procedure or surgery.

genioplasty: see *chin implantation.*

geometric broken-line closure: a scar revision technique in which a straight scar is given a new, irregular incision that is much less noticeable.

glycolic acid: an alpha hydroxy acid derived from sugar cane.

Gore-Tex™: see *expanded polytetrafluoroethylene*.

helix: the rolled-up edge that forms the outer frame of the auricle of the ear.

hematoma: a pooling of blood under the skin.

hernia: a weakness or rupture in the wall of an organ through which tissues protrude.

herniated fat: as it pertains to the eyelid, fat that protrudes through weakened muscle in the lower and/or upper lid.

herpes simplex virus (HSV): an infection which primarily causes blisters around the mouth.

humectant: a substance that attracts and retains moisture.

hyaluronic acid: an acid occurring naturally in skin tissues that can be used commercially as an injectable implant to fill fine wrinkles and facial lines.

hybrid fillers: a soft tissue filler, a blend of microscopic plastic beads and human collagen.

hydroquinone: a topical agent that blocks the formation of pigments in the skin; used to diminish freckles and other hypopigmented areas.

hypercorrection: relating to otoplasty; the condition of an ear being too close to the head after surgery.

hyperpigmentation: excess color in the skin.

hypertrophic scar: overdeveloped scars that may be thick, red, and ropey.

hypertrophy: increase in size or number of cells resulting in growth of tissue.

hypoallergenic: not likely to cause an allergic reaction.

hypopigmentation: too little color in the skin.

hypopigmented scar: scar with no pigmentation which appears white.

incision: a cut made through the skin with a knife or laser during a surgical procedure.

incisors: in humans, the four upper and lower front teeth.

injectable filler: a substance that can be injected to improve the skin's appearance cosmetically.

injectable microimplant: a substance, often containing tiny beads to provide bulk and stimulate collagen production, that is used to improve the skin's appearance cosmetically.

intense pulsed light (IPL): see *photorejuvenation*.

intraoral: inside the mouth.

intravenous (IV): inside a vein.

invasive surgery: a surgical procedure that involves making an incision or incisions and exposing internal tissues or organs.

IPL (intense pulsed light): see *photorejuvenation*.

IV: see *intravenous*.

keloid: a raised, thick, irregular scar caused by excessive tissue growth at the site of an incision or wound.

keratin: Protein found in hair, nails, and the outer layers of skin.

keratosis: a buildup of keratin—the hard protein in skin, nails, and hair—on the upper layer of skin. See also *actinic keratosis*.

lactic acid: an alpha hydroxy acid derived from milk.

laser: the acronym for *light amplification by stimulated emission of radiation*; a specialized high-energy light beam.

laser lip rejuvenation: a procedure using a laser to smooth the lips.

laser skin rejuvenation: a procedure using a laser to vaporize upper skin layers.

lateral browlift: see *temporal browlift*.

light peel: a chemical peel involving the skin's superficial layers to reduce skin irregularities such as freckles, age spots, fine lines, and wrinkles.

lip advancement: a form of surgical lip augmentation that elevates and reshapes the inner lip lining.

lip augmentation: a medical procedure using injections or surgical implantation to smooth, fill out, reshape, and enhance the lips.

lip lift procedure: to remove a strip of skin beneath the nose, shortening the distance between the nasal columella and the upper lip.

lipid-soluble: able to dissolve in oil.

liposuction: the removal of body fat using a suction device.

lobe, lobule: the fleshy lower portion of the ear.

local anesthetic: a drug that blocks pain sensations in a region of the body.

lop ear: a type of constricted ear in which the top is folded down and forward and the concha is at a right angle to the head; also called *bat ear*.

macrotia: an abnormal largeness of the ear.

malar: pertaining to the cheek.

managed-care anesthesia: office-based anesthesia, delivered by IV.

medium peel: a chemical peel that removes more skin layers than a light peel and is more effective in reducing the appearance of skin irregularities.

melanin: skin pigment.

melasma: dark discoloration of the skin.

mentoplasty: see *chin implantation*.

metabolism rate: the pace at which your body absorbs and processes nutrients.

methylparaben: see *parabens*.

microdermabrasion: removing dead skin cells to smooth the skin by "sanding" the face with fine granules or crystals.

micropigmentation: tattooing; "permanent makeup."

microtia: an abnormal smallness of the ear.

midface lift: cosmetic surgery to raise and reposition the soft tissues between the eyes and mouth.

midface suspension: procedure to lift the cheek pads with suture loops attached at the temples.

migration: movement of implanted materials away from the implant site.

milia: plural of *milium*, a small whitish bead in the skin due to a clogged sebaceous gland.

mineral oil: oil derived from a mineral source, often petroleum.

minimal-incision browlift: see *endoscopic browlift*.

mini-midface lift: see *SOOF lift*.

Myobloc™: see *Botox*.

myxedema: severe untreated hypothyroidism.

nasolabial fold: a furrow between the wing of the nose and the lip. See also *melolabial fold*.

necrosis: tissue or cell death.

nerve block anesthesia: deeper, more targeted injection of anesthetic into tissue containing sensory nerves.

nonablative laser: a skin-resurfacing device that passes through outer tissue to exfoliate and stimulate collagen production.

noncomedogenic: not likely to block the pores or cause acne lesions (*comedones*).

occlusive: physically preventing loss of moisture from the skin.

oral retinoid: medications used to treat skin conditions such as acne or psoriasis.

orbicularis: around the eye.

otoplasty: plastic surgery to reconstruct or cosmetically improve the ear.

PABA (P-aminobenzoic acid): a substance added to lotions and creams to screen out ultraviolet rays.

palpability: the quality of being tangible (able to be felt).

parabens (butyl-, ethyl-, methyl-, propyl-): cosmetic preservatives used commonly in the United States; derived from benzoic acid, found naturally in balsamic substances.

Parsol 1789™: a sunscreen ingredient that absorbs ultraviolet rays.

petrolatum: a semisolid mixture derived from petroleum and used in skin oils and ointments.

phenol: also called *carbolic acid*; a chemical used in deep peels to minimize the effects of sun damage and wrinkling.

photoaging: skin damage caused by the sun.

photorejuvenation: use of intense pulsed light (IPL) to reduce unsightly signs of aging on the skin like brown spots, broken capillaries, rosacea, and dull complexion.

plastic surgeon: a medical doctor who specializes in reducing scarring and disfigurement from accidents, birth defects, and diseases. A *cosmetic plastic surgeon* specializes in aesthetic improvement of the face and body via surgery.

physical sunscreen: sun protection ingredients that reflect ultraviolet rays.

polymer: a material composed of giant molecules made up of smaller molecules; sometimes considered synonymous with *plastic*, a polymer can be made of organic materials, such as rubber or cellulose.

porcine collagen: a connective tissue protein derived from pigs and used in injection form to help correct facial wrinkles.

pressure therapy: in scar revision, a technique in which a pressure bandage is worn over time to reduce a scar.

pretrichial incision: an incision near the hairline.

procerus: a muscle extending from the upper nose to the lower forehead that functions to wrinkle the upper nose.

propylene glycol: a synthetic preservative used in numerous substances, including skin products and antifreeze.

propylparaben: see *parabens*.

Renova™: see *tretinoin*.

Restylane™: see *hyaluronic acid*.

Retin-A™: see *tretinoin*.

retinoid: a vitamin A derivative used to treat skin conditions and for other medical applications.

rhinoplasty: cosmetic or reconstructive surgery of the nose.

rosacea: chronic inflammation and redness of the cheeks, nose, chin, forehead, or eyelids.

salicylic acid: an antimicrobial substance found in wintergreen, sweet birch, and other plants; used to make aspirin and also to remove outer skin layers.

scapha, scaphoid fossa: the scooped-out area near the edge of the ear.

sclera: the white of the eye.

sebum: a natural oil found in the skin, secreted by the sebaceous glands.

sedation: calming or rendering a patient unconscious with a sedative, a medicine that promotes tranquility and sometimes sleep.

septoplasty: a surgical procedure in which the nasal septum is straightened.

seroma: a collection of sterile body fluid beneath the skin.

shell ear: a condition of the ear in which the fold of the helix and other natural folds and creases are missing.

silicone: a synthetic polymer with hundreds of applications, often used in implants.

skin flap: tissues being transferred from one part of the body to another, including skin and underlying fat, nerves, blood vessels, and muscle.

skin graft: a thin layer of healthy skin that, once transplanted, interacts with the surrounding tissues to form a new blood supply.

skin resurfacing: removal of the outer layer or layers of skin using abrasion, chemicals, or lasers.

solar elastosis: sun-induced skin changes.

SOOF: suborbicularis (under the eye) fat.

SOOF lift: a surgical procedure that removes or redistributes suborbicularis fat to smooth the cheek area beneath the eyes.

SPF: see *sun protection factor*.

spider veins: small clusters of visible red, blue, or purple veins.

Stahl's ear: an abnormal ear formation in which the helix is flattened and the auricle's upper edge is pointed; sometimes called Spock's ear or Vulcan ear.

steroids: see *cortical steroids*.

stratum corneum: the top layer of the skin, composed of toughened, scaly cells.

subcutaneous: under the skin.

subperiosteal lift: a facelift that provides a vertical lift to the soft tissues of the face.

sun protection factor (SPF): a number assigned to sunscreen products that indicates how long its protection lasts; the higher the number, the better the protection.

sunscreen, sunblock: a topical lotion, cream, or gel that prevents ultraviolet rays from penetrating the skin.

suture bridging: a complication of otoplasty in which permanent sutures can be seen through the skin.

sutures: surgical stitches.

suture loops: loops of sutures used to lift tissue.

synthetic: human-made.

TCA: see *trichloroacetic acid.*

telephone ear: an abnormal condition of the ear in which the top and bottom of the auricle stick out farther than the rest of the ear.

temporal browlift: a type of forehead lift using small diamond-shaped incisions at the hairline on either side of the forehead.

thermoplasty, Thermage™, ThermaCool TC™, ThermaLift™: a mild skin-tightening procedure using a radiofrequency-generating device to apply intense heat to the underlying dermis while bursts of cryogen spray cool the outer skin layers.

tiplasty: a surgical procedure to reshape the tip of the nose.

titanium dioxide: a substance used in some sunscreens and other products to protect the skin from the sun and other irritants.

topical anesthetic: a local anesthetic applied externally.

transconjunctival incision: a surgical cut made on the inside of the lower eyelid.

transcutaneous: through the skin.

tretinoin: topical vitamin A derivative that exfoliates, stimulates collagen production, and evens out skin pigments; available by prescription as Retin-A™ and Renova™.

trichophytic incision: incision made a few millimeters inside the hairline.

trichloroacetic acid (TCA): a substance used in a chemical peel to remove outer layers of skin for correction of surface wrinkles, blemishes, and pigmentation problems.

twilight sleep: office-based anesthesia, delivered by IV.

ultraviolet rays (UVR): electromagnetic radiation that damages the skin and causes wrinkling, blotchiness, broken blood vessels, dryness, thinning of the skin, and skin cancer. UV-A, UV-B, and UV-C rays are ultraviolet rays distinguished by wavelength.

vascular: pertaining to blood vessels or blood supply.

vermillion: the visible part of the lip, which is typically darker than the surrounding skin.

vermillion border: the junction between the outer skin and the vermillion, or skin of the lips.

vertical lift: see *midface lift.*

W-plasty: see *geometric broken-line closure.*

wrinkle filler: collagen or another injectable substance.

Z-plasty: see *geometric broken-line closure.*

zinc oxide: an opaque skin protectant that blocks the sun's rays and also has antiseptic properties.

Zyderm™, Zyplast™: medical products containing collagen and used to fill facial lines and wrinkles.

INDEX

RESOURCES

American Academy of Facial Plastic and Reconstructive Surgery

310 South Henry Street ■ *Alexandria, VA 22314*
Phone: 703-299-9291 or 800-332-FACE
Fax: 703-299-8898 ■ *www.facial-plastic-surgery.org*

Founded in 1964, the American Academy of Facial Plastic and Reconstructive Surgery (AAFPRS) represents more than 2,700 facial plastic and reconstructive surgeons throughout the world. Among the objectives listed in their mission statement: To promote the highest quality facial plastic surgery through education, dissemination of professional information, and the establishment of professional standards. The AAFPRS is a National Medical Specialty Society of the American Medical Association. AAFPRS members are board-certified surgeons whose focus is surgery of the face, head, and neck. The Web site offers a "virtual exam"—an interactive feature that highlights the most common areas in which facial cosmetic procedures are performed. The online Patient Information Series explains procedures, helps you determine whether they're right for you, and lets you know what to expect. Also on the site are FAQs, before-and-after photos, a physician finder, and a quarterly online magazine.

American Board of Medical Specialties

1007 Church Street, Suite 404 ■ *Evanston, IL 60201-5913*
Phone: 847-491-9091 ■ *Fax: 847-328-3596* ■ *www.abms.org*

The American Board of Medical Specialties (ABMS) is an organization of twenty-four approved medical specialty boards. The intent of the certification of physicians is to provide assurance to the public that those certified by an ABMS Member Board have successfully completed an approved training program and an evaluation process assessing their ability to provide quality patient care in the specialty. This Web site explains how specialists are trained and certified; it also offers a search feature for finding certified physicians.

American Society for Aesthetic Plastic Surgery

11081 Winners Circle ■ *Los Alamitos, CA 90720*
Phone: 888-ASAPS-11 (physician referrals) ■ *www.surgery.org*

Founded in 1967, ASAPS is a professional organization of plastic surgeons, certified by the American Board of Plastic Surgery, who specialize in cosmetic plastic surgery. The organization has 2,100 members in the U.S. and Canada, as well as corresponding members in many other countries. The Web site offers an "Ask an ASAPS Surgeon" feature, as well as news, updates, and consumer-oriented reports on surgical and nonsurgical procedures. The site also has a Find-a-Surgeon feature. You'll also find numerous articles and procedure descriptions, some in both English and Spanish.

American Society of Plastic Surgeons

444 East Algonquin Road ■ *Arlington Heights, IL 60005*
Phone: 847-228-9900; 888-4-PLASTIC, 888-475-2784 (physician referrals)
www.plasticsurgery.org

The American Society of Plastic Surgeons (ASPS) is the largest plastic surgery specialty organization in the world. Founded in 1931, the society is composed of board-certified plastic surgeons who perform cosmetic and reconstructive surgery. The mission of ASPS is to advance quality care to plastic surgery patients by encouraging high standards of training, ethics, physician practice, and research in plastic surgery. The society advocates for patient safety, such as encouraging its members to operate in surgical facilities that have passed rigorous external review of equipment and staffing. The society works in concert with the Plastic Surgery Educational Foundation, founded in 1948, which supports research and educational programs for plastic surgeons. On the society's Web site are FAQs, a history of plastic surgery, a surgeon finder, capsule descriptions of procedures, patient profiles, a photo gallery, and cost information.

American Board of Plastic Surgery

Seven Penn Center
1635 Market Street, Suite 400 ■ *Philadelphia, PA 19103-2204*
Phone: 215-587-9322 ■ *Fax: 215-587-9622* ■ *www.abplsurg.org*

The mission of the American Board of Plastic Surgery is to promote safe, ethical, efficacious plastic surgery to the public by maintaining high standards for the education, examination, and certification of plastic surgeons as specialists and subspecialists. Primarily for physicians, the board's Web site includes FAQs explaining how doctors become board-certified and describing differences among licensure, certification, and accreditation.

American Academy of Cosmetic Surgery

Cosmetic Surgery Information Service
737 North Michigan Avenue, Suite 820 ■ *Chicago, IL 60611*
Phone: 312-981-6760 ■ *www.cosmeticsurgery.org*

Formed in 1985, the American Academy of Cosmetic Surgery (AACS) represents practitioners of medical disciplines including dermatology, ophthalmology, otorhinolaryngology, plastic and reconstructive surgery, oral and maxillofacial surgery, general surgery, and others. The AACS is the nation's largest organization representing cosmetic surgeons. The Academy's purpose is to maintain a membership of medical and dental professionals who participate in postgraduate medical education opportunities, specifically in cosmetic surgery, so that the public is assured of receiving consistently high-quality medical and dental care. The Academy's Web site offers assistance finding and choosing a surgeon, describes procedures and their risks, explains what to do before surgery, and helps you determine whether you're a good candidate.

American Society for Laser Medicine and Surgery

2404 Stewart Avenue ■ *Wausau, WI 54401*
Phone: 715-845-9283 ■ *Fax: 715-848-2493*
E-mail: information©aslms.org ■ *www.aslms.org*

Founded in 1981 to educate both physicians and the lay public, the society maintains a Web site with public health information that includes an introduction to and history of lasers, online referral service, standards of practice, FAQs, and links to member Web sites.

American Academy of Dermatology

P.O. Box 4014 ■ *Schaumburg, IL 60168-4014*
Phone: 866-503-7546 ■ *Fax: 847-330-0050* ■ *www.aad.org*

The American Academy of Dermatology (AAD) is the nation's largest dermatologic association. With a membership of more than 13,700, it represents virtually all practicing dermatologists in the United States. Public information on the Web site includes current and archived issues of the AAD's consumer magazine *Dermatology Insights,* free online pamphlets on surgical and nonsurgical cosmetic procedures, help in finding a dermatologist, and other consumer and patient resources.

AAD's AgingSkinNet, at www.skincarephysicians.com, offers descriptions and FAQs on treatment and management of skin conditions such as acne, aging skin, skin cancer, rosacea, eczema, actinic keratoses, and psoriasis treatments, and before-and-after photos.

American Skin Association, Inc.

346 Park Avenue South, 4th Floor ■ *New York, NY 10010*
Phone: 800-499-SKIN or 212-889-4858 ■ *Fax: 212-889-4959*
E-mail: info@skinassn.org ■ *www.americanskin.org*

The American Skin Association is a patient-advocacy group that supports research and education on skin disorders. Annual membership is $25 and includes the quarterly newsletter *SKINFacts,* educational brochures on specific skin disorders; notices of public forums and meetings; and invitations to events. Free educational pamphlets are published each year on topics ranging from *Melanoma: The Deadliest of Skin Diseases* to *Outdoor Sports and Your Skin.*

U.S. National Library of Medicine

8600 Rockville Pike ■ *Bethesda, MD 20894*
www.nlm.nih.gov ■ *www.nlm.nih.gov/medlineplus*

The National Library of Medicine Web site indexes articles (primarily for scientists and health professionals) from more than 3,500 medical journals. MedlinePlus is consumer oriented and includes information on more than 650 topics (conditions, diseases, and wellness), drug information, a medical encyclopedia and dictionary, news, provider directories, and other resources.

eMedicine, Inc.

1004 Farnam Street, Suite 300 ■ Omaha, NE 68102
Phone: 402-341-3222 ■ www.emedicine.com

Though created for an audience of health professionals, the eMedicine Web site includes informative descriptions of hundreds of procedures. Launched in 1996, the site is the most comprehensive source of information available free online about procedures, risks, side effects, anesthesia, preparation for surgery, follow-up, expectations, and other pertinent information. Nearly 10,000 physician authors and editors contribute to the eMedicine Clinical Knowledge Base, which contains articles on 7,000 diseases and disorders. The site also contains nearly 6,500 pages of patient information.

American Board of Facial Plastic and Reconstructive Surgery

115C South St. Asaph Street ■ Alexandria, VA 22314
Phone: 703-549-3223 ■ Fax: 703-549-3357
E-mail: tshill@abfprs.org ■ www.abfprs.org

This organization's mission is improving the quality of facial plastic surgery available to the public by measuring the qualifications of candidate surgeons against certain rigorous standards. To be considered for membership, a physician must have completed a residency program, have been in practice a minimum of two years, have 100 operative reports accepted by a peer review committee, successfully pass an eight-hour written and oral examination, hold the appropriate licensure, and adhere to the ABFPRS Code of Ethics.

UCLA Patient Learning Series

UCLA Medical Center
10833 Le Conte Avenue ■ Los Angeles, CA 90095-6923
Phone: 800-UCLA-MD1, 800-825-2631
www.healthcare.ucla.edu/pls/ageskin.htm

Patient Learning Series articles summarize the latest medical approaches to diagnosis and treatment; they explain key terms and emphasize things individuals can do to help themselves.

Johns Hopkins Cosmetic Center at Green Springs Station

10755 Falls Road, Suite 420 ■ Lutherville, MD 21093
Phone: 410-583-7180 ■ E-mail: cosmeticsurgery@jhmi.edu
www.hopkinscosmeticsurgery.org

The Web site includes comprehensive illustrated articles about numerous cosmetic surgical and nonsurgical procedures, including chemical peels, eyelid surgery, facelifts, liposuction, rhinoplasty, endoscopic procedures, and forehead lifts.

Cosmetic, Toiletry, and Fragrance Association

1101 17th Street, NW, Suite 300 ■ Washington, D.C. 20036-4702
Phone: 202-331-1770 ■ Fax: 202-331-1969

The association supports the cosmetic, toiletry, and fragrance industries and also coordinates educational activities and supports public service programs. CTFA Online includes an Infobase of consumer information including a buyer's guide.

www.cosmeticscop.com

13075 Gateway Drive, Suite 160 ■ Seattle, WA 98168
Phone: 206-444-1616 ■ Fax: 206-444-1626

This Web site includes a comprehensive dictionary of cosmetic ingredients compiled by Paula Begoun, author of *Don't Go to the Cosmetics Counter without Me.*

U.S. Food and Drug Administration

5600 Fishers Lane ■ Rockville, MD 20857-0001
Phone: 888-INFO-FDA, 888-463-6332 ■ www.fda.gov

The FDA Web site includes comprehensive information on all the substances and activities the agency regulates, including cosmetics, implant materials, cosmetic procedures, medications, and more.

ABOUT THE AUTHORS

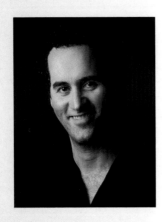

Every day I receive tremendous satisfaction in knowing that the relationships I have developed with my patients will last a lifetime. I enjoy educating patients and being educated by them.

— Dr. Jon Mendelsohn

JON MENDELSOHN, M.D., is a facial plastic surgeon in private practice in Cincinnati, Ohio. He is medical director of the Advanced Cosmetic Surgery & Laser Center. He is also co-author of *The Non-Surgical Facelift Book—A Guide to Facial Rejuvenation* (Addicus Books, 2003).

Dr. Mendelsohn received a Bachelor of Science degree in molecular biology from Syracuse University. He attended medical school at the State University of New York Health Science Center, Syracuse, and completed a residency there in otolaryngology, head and neck surgery.

Dr. Mendelsohn is board-certified by the American Board of Facial Plastic and Reconstructive Surgery and the American Board of Otolaryngology—Head and Neck Surgery. He is a fellow of the American Academy of Facial Plastic and Reconstructive Surgery, American College of Surgeons, and the American Academy of Otolaryngology—Head and Neck Surgery.

Dr. Mendelsohn is a member of the American Academy of Facial Plastic and Reconstructive Surgery's committees on multimedia and new technologies and devices. He is a national trainer in the use of Botox and Restylane and a regional trainer in the use of autologous platelet gels. He has presented nationally at conferences on facial plastic surgery and has authored numerous papers and publications on facial plastic surgery.

Dr. Mendelsohn may be reached through his Web site: **www.351face.com.**

WILLIAM TRUSWELL, M.D., is a facial plastic surgeon in private practice in Northampton, Massachusetts. He is medical director of the Aesthetic Laser and Cosmetic Surgery Center, which he founded in 1976. He is also co-author of *The Non-Surgical Facelift Book—A Guide to Facial Rejuvenation* (Addicus Books, 2003).

Dr. Truswell received a Bachelor of Science degree from Hobart College, Geneva, New York. He graduated from the University of Medicine and Dentistry of New Jersey and completed a residency in otolaryngology and facial plastic and reconstructive surgery at the University of Connecticut School of Medicine.

Dr. Truswell is board-certified by the American Board of Facial Plastic and Reconstructive Surgery (ABFPRS) and the American Board of Otolaryngology. He is a fellow of the American College of Surgeons, the American Academy of Facial Plastic and Reconstructive Surgery, the American Academy of Cosmetic Surgery, the American Academy of Otolaryngology—Head and Neck Surgery, the American Society for Head and Neck Surgery, and the American Academy of Laser Medicine Surgery.

He currently serves on the board of directors for the American Academy of Facial Plastic and Reconstructive Surgery, and is an oral examiner for the ABFPRS.

Dr. Truswell is a clinical instructor in facial plastic surgery in the Division of Otolaryngology, Department of Surgery, University of Connecticut School of Medicine. He is also a medical consultant to Atrium Medical Corporation Advanta for ePTFE facial soft tissue implants. He is the designer of the Truswell Insertion Instrument for soft tissue implants, manufactured by Marina Medical Corporation.

Dr. Truswell writes articles on facial plastic and reconstructive surgery in medical specialty journals, consults with other professionals for books on facial plastic surgery, and he lectures at facial plastic surgery meetings throughout the country. He has also presented a paper at the Royal College of Surgeons in London, and was a guest lecturer at an annual meeting of the Canadian Academy of Facial Plastic and Reconstructive Surgery.

Dr. Truswell may be reached through his Web site: **www.truswellplasticsurg.com.**

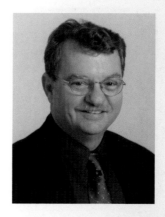

When you are in the surgeon's office, you must be the most important person to the doctor and his/her staff. This will mark the difference between a good result and an excellent result.

— *William Truswell, M.D.*

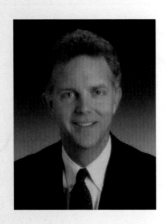

My patients want to look better. The person they see in the mirror doesn't reflect the vibrant, happy person they are. In the last decade, cosmetic procedures have become longer lasting, more natural looking, and the recovery time is faster.

— *Kriston Kent, M.D.*

KRISTON J. KENT, M.D., F.A.C.S., is the medical director of Aesthetic Surgery Specialists of Naples, Florida. Dr. Kent serves as chairman of the Florida Board of Medicine Surgical Care Committee. He is a vice president of the American Academy of Facial Plastic and Reconstructive Surgery and sits on their Board of Directors. Dr. Kent also sits on the American Board of Facial Plastic and Reconstructive Surgery Board of Directors and serves as an oral examiner for the American Board of Facial Plastic Surgery.

Dr. Kent graduated cum laude from the University of Alabama School of Medicine, where he was chapter president of Alpha Omega Alpha, the medical honor society comprised of the top ten percent of medical students. He completed his five-year residency in head and neck surgery at the University of Florida and his fellowship training in facial plastic surgery through the American Academy of Facial Plastic and Reconstructive Surgery in Cincinnati, Ohio.

Dr. Kent was appointed to the Florida Board of Medicine by Governor Jeb Bush in 2001 and was recently elected vice chairman of the Board of Medicine. Dr. Kent has dual board certifications by the American Board of Facial Plastic and Reconstructive Surgery and the American Board of Otolaryngology—Head and Neck Surgery.

Dr. Kent is regularly asked to speak and teach at national and international meetings. In 2003 he was guest lecturer for the Austral/Asian Academy of Facial Plastic and Reconstructive Surgery. Dr. Kent is a leading speaker on endoscopic facial surgery and autologous healing factors. He is a clinical associate at the University of Florida School of Medicine in facial plastic surgery.

In addition to co-authoring *Your Complete Guide to Facial Cosmetic Surgery*, he is featured in the book *The Beauty Makers*.

Dr. Kent may be reached through his Web sites at
www.naplesface.com and **www.naplesspecialists.com.**

CONSUMER HEALTH TITLES
FROM ADDICUS BOOKS

Visit our online catalog at www.AddicusBooks.com

After Mastectomy—Healing Physically $14.95
and Emotionally

Cancers of the Mouth and Throat—A Patient's Guide $14.95
to Treatment

Cataracts—A Patient's Guide to Treatment $14.95

Colon & Rectal Cancer—A Patient's Guide $14.95
to Treatment

Coping with Psoriasis—A Patient's Guide $14.95
to Treatment

Coronary Heart Disease—A Guide $15.95
to Diagnosis and Treatment

Exercising Through Your Pregnancy $17.95

The Fertility Handbook—A Guide $14.95
to Getting Pregnant

The Healing Touch—Keeping the Doctor/Patient $9.95
Relationship Alive Under Managed Care

LASIK—A Guide to Laser Vision Correction $14.95

Living with P.C.O.S.—Polycystic Ovarian Syndrome $14.95

Lung Cancer—A Guide to Treatment & Diagnosis $14.95

The Macular Degeneration Source Book $14.95

The Non-Surgical Facelift Book—A Guide $19.95
to Facial Rejuvenation Procedures

Overcoming Postpartum Depression and Anxiety $14.95

A Patient's Guide to Dental Implants $14.95

Prescription Drug Addiction—The Hidden Epidemic $15.95

Prostate Cancer—A Patient's Guide to Treatment $14.95

Simple Changes: The Boomer's Guide to a $9.95
Healthier, Happier Life

A Simple Guide to Thyroid Disorders $14.95

Straight Talk About Breast Cancer—From Diagnosis $14.95
to Recovery

The Stroke Recovery Book—A Guide $14.95
for Patients and Families

The Surgery Handbook—A Guide $14.95
to Understanding Your Operation

Understanding Lumpectomy—A Treatment Guide $14.95
for Breast Cance

Understanding Parkinson's Disease—A Self-Help Guide $14.95

Your Complete Guide to Facial Cosmetic Surgery $19.95

Organizations, associations, corporations, hospitals, and other groups may qualify for special discounts when ordering more than 24 copies. For more information, please contact the Special Sales Department at Addicus Books. Phone (402) 330-7493. Email: info@AddicusBooks.com

TO ORDER BOOKS

Please send:

_____ copies of _____ at _____ each

Total _____

Nebraska residents add 6.5% sales tax _____

Shipping/Handling _____

$4.00 for first book _____

$1.10 for each additional book _____

_____ TOTAL ENCLOSED _____

Shipping Information:

Name_____

Address _____

City_____ State_____ Zip _____

Payment Information:

☐ Visa   ☐ Mastercard   ☐ American Express

Credit card number _____

_ration date _____

_____

Order by credit card, personal check, or money order.

Send to:

Addicus Books
P.O. Box 45327
Omaha, NE 68145

Order TOLL FREE:
800-352-2873

or online at

www.AddicusBooks.com

167